CUTTING A PATH

THE POWER OF PURPOSE, DISCIPLINE, AND DETERMINATION

Dr. Sheri Dewan, MD, MS, FAANS

BROWN BOOKS
PUBLISHING GROUP

Cutting a Path
The Power of Purpose, Discipline, and Determination

Brown Books Publishing Group
Dallas, TX / New York, NY
www.BrownBooks.com
(972) 381-0009

A New Era in Publishing®

Publisher's Cataloging-In-Publication Data

Names: Dewan, Sheri, author.
Title: Cutting a path : the power of purpose, discipline, and determination / by Dr. Sheri Dewan, MD, MS, FAANS.
Description: Dallas, TX ; New York, NY : Brown Books Publishing Group, [2023] | Includes bibliographical references.
Identifiers: ISBN: 9781612546209 (hardcover) | LCCN: 2022949614
Subjects: LCSH: Dewan, Sheri. | Neurosurgeons--United States--Biography. | Women surgeons—United States-- Biography. | Indian women physicians--United States--Biography. | Work-life balance. | Discrimination in medical care. | LCGFT: Autobiographies. | BISAC: BIOGRAPHY & AUTOBIOGRAPHY / Medical.
Classification: LCC: RD592.9.D49 A3 2023 | DDC: 617.48092--dc23

ISBN 978-1-61254-620-9
LCCN 2022949614

Printed in Canada
10 9 8 7 6 5 4 3 2 1

For more information or to contact the author, please go to
www.DrSheriDewan.com

For my children Amara, Mia, and Jai.
May your dreams be limitless.

"Keep your eyes on the prize."
—Alice Wine, civil rights activist

Table of Contents

Foreword

Rarely does talent bestow its graces on one individual in multiple areas. Dr. Sheri Dewan is one of those talents. I have walked the same path as Dr. Dewan—becoming a neurosurgeon and eventually becoming the first woman appointed as a chair of neurosurgery in the United States. Like her, I have balanced the roles of wife, mother, daughter, and surgeon, and I can attest to the complexity of that balancing act.

In these pages, Dr. Dewan shares her most private thoughts while taking us along on her life's journey. Her writing allows us front-row seats into the mind of a neurosurgeon. I know these stories up close and personally, yet I found myself turning each page anxious for the next because these stories reflect the scope of the tragedy and triumph we deal with daily. Her prose allows us that insight, and her honesty is uncomfortable. In baring her soul, she urges the reader to think about issues beyond what is medically important and touches on a neurosurgeon's deepest fears and conundrums.

Dr. Dewan is not always the hero, but the reader feels reassured that she cares deeply for her patients and her family and is always trying to do more. She not only accurately describes the problems we face as neurosurgeons, but her questions also reflect issues many women and men in stressful jobs face: trying to navigate personal challenges, family obligations, and careers where so many depend on us. Her dialogue echoes what so many of us have felt, and her writing helps us better understand these fears.

Dr. Karin Muraszko

Julian T. Hoff Professor and Chair of Neurosurgery,
University of Michigan

Introduction

Every part of the tiger is designed for the hunt. Her stripes, of course, provide camouflage in the dense jungle. Though her sense of smell is better than a human's, that isn't the tiger's best asset. She will wait for the sounds of prey nearby with her perfectly designed ears before committing to the hunt. Beyond the brief training from her mother, everything a tiger does is based on instinct and evolution. There is precision in her steps, careful not to disturb the delicate foliage around her, the pads of her feet helping her move her heavy body with stealth. She will spend minutes carefully tracking and stalking, positioning herself close to the target while waiting for the opportune moment to strike. She will get within twenty to thirty feet, making a tremendous jump or a lunge in which she might briefly reach a speed of fifty miles per hour, attacking with total surprise. She might swipe with her retractable five-inch claws, holding on to the animal as it tries to escape. Antelope and deer can kick, so her belly skin is loose to protect her vulnerable spots. The vulnerabilities she has are a closely kept secret. Her weaknesses, whatever they may be, are hidden behind five-inch claws and three-inch canine teeth, all wrapped up in sinewy muscle.

I didn't have millennia of physical evolution to become a neurosurgeon. Being able to drill open a cranium and cut into a brain without harming it, operating with understanding and finesse, isn't a particular result of human development but a learned trait.

My patient's eyes were taped closed, and the ventilator wheezed its mechanical breaths in a steady, humming rhythm. Next to her was a tree of IV bags, packed red blood cells, plasma, and intravenous fluids to keep her body in equilibrium. The bags were joined into a port, which fed through a line into the cannula taped to her arm; almost as if she was tethered to balloons held at her sides.

I had willed myself into shape for this exact moment. I had hunted down the aneurysm, stalking delicately, not through jungle underbrush, but through the dura—the tough membrane just under the skull that protects the brain and spinal cord—until the artery came into view. Now I was ready to clip the aneurysm between the tiny jaws of the metal clip applier. As soon as it was clipped, I was in a race to get the patient off the anesthesia machine by getting the dura closed, the titanium plates screwed into the skull, and the scalp stitched—ideally avoiding a dreaded complication. I fought against the seizing tension in my hands, cramping from hours of tiny, intricate movements while pinching small metal tools. Five hours of surgery, the chill of climate control set to the requisite sixty-five degrees, the cold wrapping around us like a surgical drape. Already the stiffness threatened to turn my fingers into claws. Neurosurgeons can't get flustered. We can't get nervous. There is only one job: fixing the brain.

Left hand pull straight. Right hand turn loop. Right hand pull through. Deep breath. I tied off the last suture with a one-handed surgeon's knot.

I inspected the closure for any gaps, any potential areas of leakage. Clean, closed *tight tight tight*, as Dr. Cahill had instructed me almost ten years earlier. I was satisfied. "I'm done. Procedure as stated." I snapped off my white latex gloves.

The anesthesiologist called out, "Time: 22:05."

My outer layer gloves joined a mobile garbage can on wheels filled with surgical debris: blue drapes and towels with blood pooling in the creases. The surgical tables resembled a battlefield: scissors lay with tips pointing upwards, the tray of aneurysm clips open, some unused while others were marked with the stamps of blood on the blades—perfect red ovals where my gloved fingers pressed against the metal handle. Each aneurysm clip with its unique use: straight, curved, bent, angled with the colors of metallic purple, metallic blue, silver, and gold.

Though my fingers were still cold and stiff, I slowly unscrewed each pin that held her skull in the metal frame and rested her head in my freshly gloved palms. The scrub nurse rushed to attach the head of the bed, then she cleansed the patient's skin with hydrogen peroxide. It's important to remove any visible signs of blood before the family sees the patient. Doctors may be hardened to the sight of blood, the shocks of anatomy; even then, when you're not in the role of surgeon, it doesn't matter how much you've seen—when it's your loved one, it's a cut you feel deeply.

I applied the tight packing to avoid post surgical swelling, turning the cotton wrap onto her scalp, with each pass covering another section of the incision and her hair. I had made a minimal shave, taking only what I needed to clear a space for the incision. Women are particularly sensitive about their appearance. Those in neurosurgery call this scar a mark of beauty. Though it fades, though it often gets hidden by the growth of hair, the lines remain, irrevocably woven into the fabric of one's skin.

I was in my office on my twenty-four-hour on-call shift the day before when Ruth, my patient, arrived in the emergency room at our suburban hospital on the outer rim of the greater Chicago metropolitan area. I got the page from the ER physician and headed downstairs from my office to get her story, nodding with the details. I could predict the next lines, the uncanny familiarity of events with this particular diagnosis. I knew the blueprints of each disease, each neurological disorder, each accident—it was pattern recognition.

It had been a normal day for Ruth: a bright blue sky punctuated by birds flapping toward the horizon, a to-do list of errands. Insignificant, inconsequential daily duties. And then it happened. Ruth was overcome with a sudden, severe thunderclap headache. A throbbing pressure. She slumped forward, holding her head. The vomiting began. She lost consciousness. The ambulance arrived to transport her to the nearest hospital with neurosurgical capabilities.

A ruptured intracranial aneurysm.

It was an old foe of mine. I don't use the term lightly. Neurosurgeons generally have to be neutral, in control, inured while we follow hot on the trail of disease. The brain is not the enemy; however, ruptured aneurysms were personal to me.

When a blood vessel in the brain grows weak, it will balloon with blood, most of the time offering no warning signs it's even there. If it's caught before it ruptures, it can be clipped off to prevent bleeding out. Once it ruptures, though, it will bleed into the brain and mix with the cerebrospinal fluid the brain floats in. When blood flow to the brain is disrupted, it doesn't get to the vital tissue that needs oxygen and nutrients. This will cause a stroke.

I met Ruth, her husband, and their fifteen-year-old daughter in the ER. The odds of even making it to the hospital alive were 30 percent. She was here; she was one of the lucky ones.

I asked if she had been complaining of headaches. They each replied, adding information, looking for signs they would later regret missing.

"Yes, but she always had headaches. She had been taking Tylenol."

"We thought it was her sinuses."

"We thought she had stress. We thought she was developing migraines."

"She saw her doctor, had her blood pressure checked, had a physical, had bloodwork."

"We never suspected this."

"We were told everything was okay."

Families always ask if they should have seen the signs, if they could have done more. They carry with them a lingering guilt; the rehashing of the day, looking for moments of meaning, a moment to look back to that says if you had only seen this detail, you could have had total control over the whole situation and worked a miracle. No one can be prepared for a life-changing day or to learn how powerless we often are in preventing catastrophe. It's a moment that is attached in time with a scar, a cut so deep the mark never truly goes away.

As soon as the surgical bed was reattached, I set Ruth's wrapped head down, turning to our circulating nurse, Nicole. "Have the family meet me in the consult room," I said.

Nicole nodded. She had been an anchor of the hospital staff for over twenty years and had no doubt seen this scenario many times before. She whispered, "Is she going to make it, Dr. Dewan?"

I looked down. I didn't have to say any more to Nicole. She knew. It all depended on how she did in the next few, but critical, days.

I replayed the surgical procedure in my head with all its intricate details. After meeting with Ruth's family, I would dictate my operating procedure for the medical chart:

"Patient was pinned in three-point Mayfield head frame fixation. The overlying hair was minimally shaved, exposing the right frontotemporal region.

"A pterional incision was completed using a skin marker. She was then prepped and draped after appropriate timeout procedure.

"Following infiltration with local anesthetic, the skin incision was created.

"The galeal flap was retracted inferiorly. A retractor was placed for adequate visualization.

"Next, a craniotomy was performed in the frontotemporal location, and a small bone flap was turned and placed in saline solution.

"The dura was incised, the frontal and temporal lobes inspected.

"Two retractors were placed on the frontal and temporal poles, identifying the Sylvian fissure.

"I was able to obtain proximal control and work my way distally to find the apex of the aneurysm.

"A titanium aneurysm clip was placed."

The steps were regimented, a militaristic routine, orderly; the process necessary for a neurosurgeon. Names like Sylvian fissure—the fissure on the side of the brain that makes it look like it's been folded over—and a galeal flap—a protective layer of scalp beneath the skin—were terms as familiar as the names of my own children.

The perils of the procedure were evident going in: disability or death. I had to know every possible counterattack; be prepared, methodical, and then acclimate for any possibility: things that could go wrong, things that may go wrong, things that have gone wrong. My steps and movements were rehearsed and honed over seven years of residency training and now more than an equal number of years in neurosurgical practice.

Once Ruth was taken to the ICU, I scrubbed out by ripping off my paper surgical gown, discarding my surgical mask, and removing my surgical goggles. My thoughts strayed back to Ruth's husband and daughter, sitting in the waiting room, apprehensive and hopeful. These were not abstract emotions for me. I saw their thoughts as pulsating neurons racing through their brain, their emotions running through electrical wires up and down the spinal column. I felt them in my deepest, most ingrained hippocampal memories.

As soon as I was out of the OR, I was hit by a wave of hunger and thirst. My stomach cramped. Over five hours since I'd had my small bottle of cranberry juice—sometimes it's apple juice—both provide the extra kick I need to get through a long surgery. I ate light a few hours before the procedure to avoid fatigue from digestion. I avoided water for most of the day to ensure I wouldn't have to scrub out to use the bathroom. I learned early in my career what was needed in order to make my body work to its maximal effectiveness. My body became robotic. I turned off all the sensations, sounds, distractions, to focus on my current task. Once that task was performed, I was free to reengage.

I took a few sips of water and then made my way to Ruth's husband and daughter, who were waiting for me in the surgical consultation room. Her husband's hands were folded across his lap, his flannel shirt untucked, his jeans riding above his well-worn work boots. Her daughter's hair was jumbled into a ponytail, her face and posture seeming younger after carrying so much fear. I sat down in the chair across from them, sinking into the cushion—the first rest in over five hours. The aching that squeezed and pounded at my legs was immediately relieved. My feet, throbbing and swollen from standing in one place, tingled. My hands regained feeling after hours of numbness. But I was far from relaxed. I had to be the voice explaining the procedure in terms the family would understand. I had to calm them, but I had to keep them realistic. I had to prepare them without destroying their hope completely.

"I was able to identify and clip the aneurysm. An intraoperative angiogram was performed. It's a type of X-ray scan, using dye to evaluate the arteries, and it showed no filling inside the clip."

The daughter let out a sharp exhale, as if the air that had been trapped in her body released, as if she had been holding that wind since the start of her mother's surgery. She settled back in her seat.

"But," I continued, "there was extensive swelling. I needed to place an external drainage catheter into the brain to relieve pressure. She will likely need this for over a week. There is a chance she may require a permanent shunt—a tube that extends from the brain into the belly for drainage of spinal fluid."

The daughter tensed again. "Is the tube on the outside of the body?" she asked.

"No, this would be internal. But we need to get her through the next several days. There is a condition called vasospasm that can occur between day four and fourteen, when arteries constrict or tighten. This can lead to strokes or oxygen deprivation to certain portions of the brain." It was the news I hated to give. A vasospasm often, not always, can lead to brain death. "She is still very critical."

Ruth's husband nodded. "Thank you, Doctor. I know that you are doing everything that you can. I know how serious this is."

I was a complete stranger to them before their wife and mother entered the emergency room the day before. And now I had opened up her skull. I became responsible for the tremendous task of saving the most precious woman to them.

It's a paradoxical kind of intimacy between surgeons and patients, an intimacy between total strangers that seems initially transactional but later becomes a powerful tether that binds surgeon, patient, and family together for years to come.

We rose, her husband gripped my hand and tried to contain his emotions. The daughter stepped forward to shake my hand but then came closer.

"May I?" she asked.

She embraced me in a hug with deep warmth that filled me from the top of my head to the soles of my aching feet.

My twenty-four-hour call had come and gone while I was in surgery, so after checking on Ruth in the ICU, I headed to the locker room to change from my teal scrubs back into street clothes. I still needed to rehydrate my body.

Outside, a light dusting of snow lay on my car as if a soft feather had brushed my windshield. The night was pitch black except for the lights of the hospital that illuminated my path.

Few cars were on the road in this Chicago weather at this hour. The forecast was for one to two inches, and those who didn't need to be outside would stay indoors. As my car heated up, I sank into my seat, my body freeing itself of its tension, the seats warming away the numbness.

I turned to a Coldplay album on my playlist, upping the volume until it was loud enough to wash over me. Leave work at work, I reminded myself. I challenged myself to relax a little—and then my pager trilled.

The ICU nurse who had Ruth for the night was calling to confirm orders, being diligent, having noted a discrepancy. I was fooling myself to think that I could get Ruth off my mind for the evening. I had learned to navigate work life and home life, but work life would never be fully compartmentalized.

I wanted to hug my kids and smell their hair, to climb in bed with them and stay there for a week. I thought of my mom and wanted to call her, but the hour was late, and she would already be asleep.

The snow followed me all the way home, an entire layer covering my driveway. Inside, my house was still—calm and noiseless. It was nice to have quiet that was full and deep. I crept through the rooms, passing by where my children slept. My daughters, Amara and Mia, always wanted me to wake them when I came home at night. Sometimes I would stand in their rooms and listen to their quiet, slow breaths. I wouldn't disturb them tonight. I needed to collapse in my own bed, where my husband had been long asleep. Alex's breaths were a peaceful rhythm that I interrupted by climbing into bed next to him and burying myself under the comforter.

"How did it go?" Alex asked. He always took an interest in my cases, the people I treated.

"I got the clip on and the angio was good. She was really swollen. I'm not sure she will make it." My heart was heavy. It can't be personal. It can't be personal. It can't be personal.

"You did the best you could. Just get some rest. There is nothing you can do now." His tone was practical. Alex was right in practical terms; the best thing I could do for Ruth was rest up and prepare for the next few days ahead. Alex rolled over and wrapped his arms around me, his warmth melted the ice in my veins. And yet I couldn't sleep.

Every few minutes, I imagined the trill of my pager on the nightstand. I replayed the steps I took in Ruth's surgery. I critiqued my process, thinking I could have cauterized the muscle sooner to avoid additional blood loss. I repeated the moves, imagining how I could be more agile, nimble, and more successful in my next case. I likened this to a tiger challenging itself to be better with each hunt. This is what neurosurgeons do. We crave perfection.

We crave perfection when perhaps what we should be striving for is adaptability. That would indeed make us more tiger-like.

I envied Alex, asleep and peaceful, not having to worry about dying patients at the hospital. Life would be so much easier if I only had my family to worry about. I had enough family worry to last me a few lifetimes. I wasn't much older than Ruth's daughter that day, more than twenty years earlier, when the tables were turned, and I had been the one pacing the waiting room. Waiting for the neurosurgeon to arrive and give us news, any news. How I hung on his every word. *Please, Ruth, make it through the night.*

I blinked, and it was no longer night.

"Mommy, wake up." I was jostled with the gentle hands of my seven-year-old.

I had been dreaming of sand dunes so high that they caressed the sky. I was in Saudi Arabia, the dunes of Dhahran. The old familiarity from my childhood was there, and I smelled the sea and earth around me, when I was young and my parents could protect me from anything. So, I had slept after all. But I'd forgotten to rehydrate. My muscles felt stiff, and my mouth was dry. My head pounded.

"Are you taking us to school today? Did you come in our room last night?" Mia asked. She didn't pause between questions, and her big brown eyes took me in as she tried to get her fill of mom time.

It was 7:30 a.m. and I had overslept.

Alex already had the kids ready to leave for school.

Amara was just behind her younger sister. "Are you doing surgery today? Or are you in clinic?" Then came the multitude of questions and comments, trying to gauge if I had time for them.

Was I on-call?

Would I be home for dinner?

Would I take them to the birthday party on Saturday?

Would I go ice skating this weekend?

Did I know Mia lost a tooth at school? Mrs. Kennedy pulled it out!

Did I know Amara learned a new piece for the piano?

"I can do three cartwheels in a row!" Mia said, wanting to demonstrate her new skill down the hallway.

"Come on, guys, we are going to be late!" Alex prodded from the end of the hall, herding our kids to the garage. My son, Jai, grabbed my arm and wouldn't let go.

"My mommy!" he yelled, glaring at his sisters, daring them to come close to me. They both knew better and backed away as he impishly grinned at his temporary victory. There was a flurry of backpacks, hats, and mismatched gloves. Jai yelled, "But I need my show-and-tell!"

I grabbed the shoebox on the counter filled with dinosaurs and Lego parts. Three quick kisses and just as suddenly as the whirlwind had begun, it was gone. The house quieted again, and the din of children turned into the sound of the dog's clinking chain and my footsteps.

I logged into the hospital computer system on my laptop, hoping Ruth's CT scan had been completed. I reviewed her chart, noting lab values and any documentation from the night staff. Her brain CT showed swelling and blood inside her ventricles, which contain the cerebrospinal fluid. There were no fluid collections surrounding the brain that warranted concern. She had made it through the night without any major events.

I felt the desperation of Ruth's fifteen-year-old daughter who had clung to my words, my facial expressions. She clung to hope, the chance her mother could be "normal" again. Whole again.

I was able to save Ruth and give her back to her family—a true gift—but I knew the woman I returned to them would not be the wife and mother they had known. Recovery would be long and imperfect. Life and routines would have to be learned again. But with persistence and hope, they would find a new way forward.

The truth is that neurologic disorders steal from patients. Brain tumors, strokes, brain aneurysms, they drop patients into a dark abyss and leave them with clouded, fractured minds. They remove dreams and leave in their place the changelings hemiparesis, hemiplegia, aphasia. On top of that, neurologic disorders are messy thieves. They smash windows and break doors off hinges. They leave collateral damage. They can steal entire lives, leaving nothing but the shell of a human form.

Neurosurgeons know that a high percentage of their patients won't survive. We know that if they survive, it can be with an asterisk or with a whole new set of complications. That is the nature of the field. We attempt to do what was once thought impossible, and now it is merely improbable. Our training and skill give us something akin to a superpower. That is an incredible gift. When we succeed, we have done the miraculous; when we don't succeed, we have to push past defeat and think of new battle strategies for the next fight. We can't make it personal. But every once in a while, there is a case that gets through our laboriously constructed battlements. Every once in a while, we get the patient, the case, that hits home.

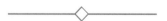

"It's not brain surgery" goes the common saying, often accompanied with an eye roll or a note of exasperation, as if to say, "Get it done, it's not that difficult." Sure, fine, but the steps it took for me to become a neurosurgeon—not the schooling and training, but the setting of goals and sticking to them and enduring even when the going gets hard—are the steps it can take for anyone to achieve a goal. It's not a matter of me saying, "If I can do it, everyone can do it," because no, not everyone has the capacity or desire to choose the life and full dedication it takes to become a neurosurgeon. Same thing with an astronaut, or a firefighter, or a restaurant chef. It took a sense of purpose, discipline, and determination to get where I did, but at its foundation, I followed my dream by carefully plotting a course and sticking to it with the focus of a mother tigress stalking dinner for her cubs. Working toward any goal from that foundation is something anyone can do.

In the course of my study of the brain and years of working on the brain, I learned not just how to cut in and operate on the most complex organ we have, but I also learned the ways in which the brain works: how it can be trained, how obstacles can be overcome, and how passion and hope and love can feed the brain, just like nutrients in soil can sustain a rainforest.

This book recounts my journey to becoming a neurosurgeon, yes, but it also shares the steps that have become mantras in my life, mantras I still use to surmount the most difficult obstacles and achieve impossible goals. My hope is that my story, and these mantras, can help you realize your own goals and dreams with tangible steps, utilizing the power of the brain and what can be achieved when we work with intention.

1

———

Go for Your Moonshot:
Capitalizing on Your Origin Story

Everyone has an origin story.

We often think of an origin story in terms of superheroes (or supervillains)—the seed that was sown, the path that forked, the crisis point that led the person to *this* life instead of *that*. The truth is that we all have a story of how we got to where we are, the inspirational moment or experience that became the driving force or the polestar. Sometimes this is a film watched at an impressionable time, or a teacher giving the golden piece of advice and encouragement—a perfect encounter of being in the right place at the right time.

Sometimes, though, an origin story involves being at the wrong place at the wrong time. Origin stories do often stem from trauma. Trauma is transformative. Trauma so acutely marks a *before* and an *after*. We would rather not have to experience it, but whether you believe in fate or coincidence or you just want to call it the Chance of Life, trauma is as old as time and will go on as long as there are living beings to experience it.

So often, trauma comes out of nowhere, inflicted upon us by an external force, rather than the summation of a series of personal choices (though trauma can come from that as well).

But what you choose to do with that trauma is key. Taking back agency is a critical step, both for mental health and for your future. Trauma, and the ensuing grief and stress, is a great force that tricks you into feeling helpless and hopeless. Stress increases the hormone cortisol, which activates our fight-or-flight responses. Trauma can lead to chronic stress, which keeps the brain in a constant state of fight-or-flight, affecting the amygdala—the fear center of the brain. Long-term stress can lead to changes within our memory centers (the hippocampus), affecting our cognition and processing. Chronic stress also increases cortisol, which leads to inflammation, and thus it can affect every organ in our body. Most importantly, it can put you at a higher risk of stroke or other neurologic diseases. Taking agency and not letting stress overwhelm you not only helps you stay on track with your goals, but is also essential for maintaining good health.

My origin story as a neurosurgeon came on a day that was as normal as the day that Ruth and her husband and daughter spent before the worst day of their collective lives. Another crystal clear but cold winter day, so many years earlier.

———◇———

My damp palms squeezed the steering wheel, heading to the suburban hospital on the outer rim of the metro Chicago area. For the fourth time, I replayed every detail of my sister's middle-of-the-night call. The call that woke me up and changed my life as I had known it.

"Sheri, it's Mom. She's really sick. You need to come to the hospital now."

I sat up in bed after a deep sleep, jarred by my sister's voice on the end of the line.

"What do you mean?" I rubbed my eyes, making sure this wasn't one of those awful dreams that you wake up from, relieved that it's over.

"They have taken her by ambulance. She was complaining of a headache, then she started vomiting and passed out." Jiji's voice hitched.

I looked around the room, at my clock, at my rumpled comforter at my waist, and the early light just beginning its creep through my window. I was indeed awake. "What did the doctors say?"

She swallowed hard, struggling to maintain composure with pressured speech. "I'm not sure what's happening. They are running tests, blood work, and they took a CT scan of her brain. Sheri, they said she has bleeding inside her brain. As if she hit her head or fell somewhere."

Bleeding in her brain. I tried to focus. What were the facts I knew? What were the details of her last few weeks?

"Did she tell you anything about hitting her head?" Jiji asked. I thought back to my most recent conversations with my mother. There had been no mention of a fall or injury of any kind. She wasn't really at the age where some people might start falling at home, but also, that wasn't my mother. Only a couple of years earlier, she'd taken me on a trek of the Annapurna range in the Himalayas, having more energy than I did on the hiking trail. The very thought of her being gravely ill didn't register with me; my mother never let illness slow her pace. Even with the slightest flu or cold virus, she pressed on, whether she was overextended or overscheduled. The woman exuded strength and power.

My sister and I had just celebrated Christmas with our parents a month earlier. Were there signs of illness I missed? Had she been complaining of headaches?

I couldn't get to the hospital fast enough.

There was minimal traffic on the roads, only my car hurtling through the empty streets of a city that otherwise throbbed with activity. I thought back to my undergraduate biology courses and neuroscience research, searching for answers. I enjoyed tackling complex problems, thriving on the methodology, feeling as bold and in control as a tiger with the information. My research project involved integrins, which are cell adhesion receptors in the brain. The integrin's particular beauty is its ability to connect or bind to the cerebral surface of the brain and thereby cause developmental acquisition and cortical layer formation—or, you could say, brain growth. But none of this knowledge could explain what had happened to my mother. I knew brain and cell development, but what did I really know about its real life applications? None of it could help me wrestle the dread I felt, the paradox of wanting to get to my mother's side as soon as I could and fearing what would happen as soon as I got there. It was the old thought experiment of Schrödinger's cat: if I didn't open the proverbial box, my mother was still both okay and not okay.

Yet there I was, driving into the hospital parking lot a few short miles from my parents' home, a hospital I had visited many times throughout my young adulthood for internist visits or signing of school forms required by my high school's sports teams. I maneuvered into an open spot and quickly reached for my down jacket and gloves. I raced for the front entrance where I was met by the perpetually cheerful hospital greeter whose purpose is to put everyone at ease. I naively bought into the possibility that things might actually be fine, that it was all potentially a misunderstanding and Jiji had been mistaken, or I'd get there, and my mom would say, "What's the big fuss?"

The greeter was calm. Friendly. Nice. That was a good thing. It had to be a good thing. But she scrolled through the computer system for what seemed an inordinate amount of time, as if she was searching the entire Project Gutenberg archives. *Alright, already, I need to see my mother.* I started to doubt the friendliness. Was it a con?

My mother is okay. My mother is not okay.

"Okay, there she is. I'll have to take you through." She then led me past the waiting room, through the first badge-in door, then the next, then the next, a monotony of wood paneling. I wondered how many more doors there could possibly be in this hospital until we stopped before a room marked with a yellow flag on the door.

Inside was my mother, lying on a stretcher, both guardrails raised. The marionette string IV lines were suspended above her, dripping their clear fluids. Her eyes were squeezed tight, brow furrowed, jaw clenched as she gripped her head.

She opened her eyes when she heard me come in.

"Hello. Hi, honey, why are you here?" she said, then immediately clutched her head again, grimacing.

Jiji and my father sat by her bedside. They were feverishly signing release forms for treatment, multiple stacks filled with medical jargon lying on my father's lap. Vials of blood with their multicolored tops rested on a metal tray next to her. Every five minutes, the beep of the blood pressure cuff marked its cycle.

My mother suddenly turned her head to vomit bile into a pink plastic basin at her chin.

"I don't . . . I don't know what's wrong with me. Why do I feel like this?"

PLEASE HELP HER, SOMEBODY DO SOMETHING, I wanted to scream at the top of my lungs to the nurse outside the door and the doctor seated at the computer outside, to anyone within earshot, to God and the whole universe. Instead, I took a long, deep breath and listened to the blood pressure cuff pulsing through its cycles and the fluids dripping from their bags. My head pounded as my heart rate skyrocketed. Pain and helplessness had settled over my father's features. Jiji's jaw was locked, her mouth a narrow line. We weren't the family that betrayed a lot of emotions, no matter what we were feeling inside. We intellectualized, rationalized, collected puzzle pieces until everything was set in its logical place.

Always, always there had been my mother to fall on when we were at our lowest. It was my mother who kept us strong by taking the reins, always knowing what to do.

Outside the door of the hospital room, a cluster of nurses were conversing in medical terms. "The family claims no trauma, no anticoagulation, non-smoker. Healthy forty-nine-year-old. We just paged Dr. Johnson, he's on his way."

Who was Dr. Johnson?

The door closed with a soft click, and we were left with my mother gripping her head and a beeping heart monitor that didn't want us to forget it was still working overtime. The machines hummed and whirred a mechanical monotony. For a while, those were the only sounds. I was woefully unprepared for the illness of a parent. The thought of illness had never entered my mind. Perhaps it was naivety, the immaturity of a young adult, or denial of an experience that would shatter one's own inner sense of stability. We'd already had our family tragedy when my grandfather was killed in a plane crash before I was born. Wasn't that more than enough for a family? Ours had lived around the world, worked hard, and thrived in our respective fields. We'd taken care to live right, be healthy, be good people. This wouldn't happen to a good person . . . would it?

My mom was gasping from pain, and my dad leaned over to kiss her hand, which was pressed against her head. He may have appeared calm, but I recognized it more as a trance-like state. In avoiding a show of emotion, he retreated somewhere far away.

Would my mom make it to her fiftieth birthday next month? Would last Christmas be the last holiday we spent as a family? Though I was in my early twenties, I still felt like the naïve child of the family, as if I needed to still be taken care of. I hadn't felt this way when I went to bed the night before, but there it was, the raw emotions seeping in.

There were so many moments of my life I expected my mom's presence. Graduations. My wedding. The meeting of her grandchildren. I thought of all the things she would teach them about life and literature. All the things she'd already taught me, and the many more lessons I'd still hoped to learn from her.

She was a lover of history and was an avid (obsessive) book reader. When Jiji or I would ask a question on any topic, her reply was always, "Look it up." We would march to the *Encyclopedia Britannica, circa 1984,* neatly placed in the cherrywood bookshelf that ran the length of our hallway and find the detailed accounting.

My mother was a political science professor at a local college who had introduced me to Sinclair's *The Jungle* and Kafka's *The Metamorphosis.* Books flooded our home, piled into bookshelves or by her bedside table, stacked in mismatched shapes and angles. She showed us how to love literature and each Saturday took Jiji and me on excursions to the local library, where we could check out five books a week. We would spend a few hours pacing the rows and stacks of steel shelves. The librarian would stamp our newest endeavors for the week and dutifully remind us, "You have ten days before late fees." By the time I was ten, I was checking out books that were well beyond my age level, as I was fascinated with the human body. I had no way of knowing what all the terminology meant, but I read every word, and I studied the pictures and diagrams faithfully.

"Another strange medical book?" Jiji asked as I brought my stack up to the counter. "My sister is so weird," she said under her breath. But my mother laughed and told me I should read whatever I was interested in.

"Leave her be. After all, your interests may seem unusual to Sheri, you know?" She cocked an eyebrow as my sister grabbed her Incan architecture guide from the librarian.

For me, the body was a puzzle to solve, a mystery to unravel. Because of my mother, I was inspired to push myself to do the hardest thing possible and succeed in it. She never met a challenge she couldn't face head-on.

"What is the hardest field in medicine?" I asked her one day.

"Oh, that's probably brain surgery," she said. "Neuroscience. It is so complex."

I nodded. "Then that's what I think I want to do."

My mother smiled. "You do whatever you want. Just do it really, really well and develop a love and passion for it."

Beyond books, my mother filled our home with her students from all ages and walks of life. She took these students on field-study trips to India to show them the life of the people and culture they were studying; it gave them a magnifying-glass view of the disparity in their fortunes. They would return transformed from their experiences.

Everyone who knew my mother was equally transformed by her. In fact, only a year before her hospitalization, she'd received the Woman of the Year award from the American Association of University Women, an organization that identifies women in the community who have made a difference through their advocacy, their research, and their passion for women's advancement in academic settings. My mother was awarded for her work in racial justice, excellence in her teaching and in her outreach, her trips with her students to India, and her tireless efforts to bring attention to the disparity of economy and opportunity for women across societies. The *Chicago Tribune* also ran a feature on her called "The Human Dynamo." The reporter visited her classrooms and came to our home for an interview.

Tireless. Unstoppable. The Human Dynamo was now throwing up bile in the hospital with bleeding in her brain.

I was startled by the knock. In fact, it was a firm rap at my mother's door, and the neurosurgeon swept into the room—bald head shining, youthful and vibrant energy even for a man in his late forties, a bowtie perfectly cinched at his neck. Dr. Douglas Johnson. Though he wasn't tall, his presence filled the room, a confidence and charisma that made me believe he held every answer and had mastered total control of this situation. Everything about him announced he was an expert in his field.

He was the first neurosurgeon I had ever met.

My father stood up. Dr. Johnson took his hand and gave it a quick shake. "Your wife is very ill. It appears that she has suffered a ruptured cerebral aneurysm, involving an artery in the brain." He then added without pausing, "Thirty percent of patients die before reaching the hospital. She was lucky to make it here alive."

So much information poured from his mouth as the words hung in the air. I had taken enough biology classes to understand what an aneurysm was, what it does to people, that it kills people. But my mother? That she was lucky to even make it to the hospital? *This is real, this is happening, this is real.* Dr. Johnson's words pinged in my brain, firing like tiny mortars. *Mom, aneurysm, lucky to be alive.* Bad, this was bad.

"We need to get a study of the arteries, called a cerebral angiogram. It needs to be done now. This will show us where the aneurysm is located and how best to treat it. I will come and speak with you after the study is completed."

And then he was out the door. He wasn't curt; it was more that he had breezed out of the room or dissolved into a puff of smoke like a wizard.

We nodded our heads in silence as a team of medical personnel rushed in and wheeled my mother to a deeper part of the hospital.

After several hours of waiting and staring at the patterned linoleum on the hospital floor, Dr. Johnson emerged from the hallway in the distance. We could see him coming, pointedly, in our direction. We stood before he entered.

"We have completed the angiogram," he said without delay. "She has a ruptured anterior communicating artery aneurysm. She will need open brain surgery so that we can place a clip on the aneurysm."

"She what . . . she needs . . . brain surgery?" my father sputtered. He shook his head, as if to ward off the facts.

"What are the risks of surgery?" I asked.

"Stroke, bleeding, infection, paralysis, neurologic deficit, and possible death."

He said the word.

She could die.

That word awakened me. That word had hovered over our heads for the last ten hours. It had circled through the stale air in the family waiting room. It had licked at the outer edges of our minds before clinging to our bones like a chill. But that chill had just been the air conditioning, I told myself. But now here it was, straight from his mouth. It was in the air, it hung, it suspended.

"How does something like this happen?" my father asked.

Dr. Johnson shrugged. "Many reasons: high blood pressure, smoking, although that doesn't seem to be your mother's case. Intracranial aneurysms can also be hereditary."

Wait, what was that? I wanted to stop him, but Dr. Johnson moved on to discussing my mother's surgery prep, and then he was gone. *Hereditary?* I looked at Jiji, and Jiji looked at me. Okay, we would address this later. For now, my mother needed to be fixed. Cured.

We put our trust in his hands that night.

That was all we could do.

A complete stranger.

My mother's organs would be viewed tonight. Her skull would be drilled, her brain investigated. A clip would be placed on a leaking artery. We saw her one last time before she was wheeled off to an unknown location.

I stood mute as the nurses rolled her bed away from us.

After six unendurable hours, Dr. Johnson met us in the waiting room, all of us limp and worn. His bald head bore a line etched by his surgical cap, his hands with marks from the latex gloves, slightly discolored from the constant pressure. He looked tired, though his youthful glow remained, albeit slightly dulled.

"The surgery has been completed. The aneurysm was identified. It was indeed leakage from the anterior communicating artery. I was able to place a titanium clip, but," he paused, "there was an arterial rupture."

"What does that mean?" I asked.

"It means that she may have had a stroke. We won't know until we can wake her up and examine her."

A stroke. My mother. A stroke.

"We will be taking several CT and MRI scans over the next few days. I also needed to place a small tube into the brain, called an external ventricular catheter. This drains spinal fluid and relieves brain pressure. Her situation is still very critical. She may be impaired due to the stroke."

Ventricular catheter. Stroke. Critical. Impaired.

"The biggest issue now is vasospasm. This is an arterial constriction that can occur beginning day four to fourteen of the rupture. It can cause blood to be cut off from critical brain structures, resulting in worsening of strokes or bleeding."

He paused, letting us digest the information. I don't know how much was actually digesting. More like reeling. The words spun around us, whipped us up like a cyclone. "Plan on her being in the hospital at least a month, that would be the best-case scenario."

He rose and gripped my father's outstretched hand in a handshake. I wanted to embrace him and feel his warmth. I wanted to tell him how deeply grateful I was that my mom was alive. But I didn't. Instead, I awkwardly shook his hand as if I was completing my first job interview. Like a kid playing at being a grown-up, I still hadn't grasped what was in store for our family and how our lives would be changed.

My heart seized when I finally saw her in the ICU, the large white mummy bandage wrapped around her head, resembling a cotton ball. The head wrapping was secured by two pieces of tape. Her skin was paper white, as if the blood had been drained out of her body. Around her mouth were the remains of adhesive tape, like two red scars left behind by a stubborn Band-Aid. I realized they were the kind of tape marks left behind when a ventilator was inserted. The tape marks were all that I needed to have the image of my mother sprawled out on a bed with a ventilator; an image I could barely comprehend and an image I couldn't shake.

She looked up at us and said, "I think there is some problem with my brain. I think that's why I'm here."

The young nurse gave us a knowing smile as she continued arranging monitors and repositioning drainage bags. One bag contained a deep red fluid, and I followed the line to my mother's skull. This must have been the external drain Dr. Johnson mentioned. It struck me—she was draining actual brain fluid.

My mother moistened her mouth to speak. "I know exactly what happened today," she said. "I was walking by some high-tension wires and then I was struck. Honey, I was struck by lightning! That's why I'm here."

My dad stepped to my mother's side. "Dear, let's just settle down. Everything is fine. We're here. You're going to be okay."

The ICU nurse was well trained and pulled my father, my sister, and me into the hallway. "This is very typical for ruptured aneurysms in this location. She will be confused. It's normal, it will get better slowly. Plus, she has likely suffered a stroke."

I didn't know what to do with that information. Normal, stroke, stroke, normal. I knew the consequences of an aneurysm, but making it through surgery, I thought she would be alright. But a stroke? Every time it came up, it completely changed the ballgame.

Three more days of waiting, of breath-holding. I thought for the first time that she could be okay, as the surgical gauze was being unwound from my mother's head. By the second turn, a perfect dime-sized circle of blood, tinged with brown, was revealed. By the third turn, the circle had bloomed, and on each consecutive pass it showed a wider, fresher, blood stain. I leapt to an absurd memory of making animations on pads of sticky notes, flipping the pages back-to-front to make the image move. A running stick figure. A setting sun. A blossoming blood stain on a surgical head wound.

My mother's bandage was off. The right side of her head was shaved, and where her hair had been, there was a line of thick staples pinching the raw flesh that would become a scar, if it healed properly. Fresh spots of blood beaded at the edges. The rest of her beautiful black hair was matted to her head, caked with blood, bone, and tissue. I was heartbroken. I was revolted.

"Great," Dr. Johnson said. "This looks good."

If that was his definition of good, I didn't want to see what his bad was. A chill rolled up my spine, and I wanted to recoil. But my mother was watching me, studying my face. "It looks good, Mom," I said, taking a step closer, trying to fix a smile for her. "It really looks like it's healing."

"Okay, then," Dr. Johnson said, "we will keep monitoring her, see how she progresses."

But by the end of the day, though she had been receiving round-the-clock care in the ICU, my mother became more confused and slurred her words.

"Why is my head hurting, Sheri?" she asked, though my name came out more like *Schlurri*.

I reached over to touch her arm. "Are you okay, Mom? Do you want me to call someone to come in?"

"My head is starting to throb. Why won't Maa get the fans in here?"

The nurse took my mother's pulse, then asked for her to raise her arms, push and pull with strength.

I realized my hands were balled into fists; my palms sweaty.

The nurse furrowed her brow. "Let me just step out a minute, okay?"

I heard her ask the secretary to page Dr. Johnson, who came to assess her within thirty minutes. He was dressed in his scrubs—no bowtie this time—as if he'd just come from the operating room.

"Looks like a vasospasm could be starting. Get a STAT CT brain, adjust the blood pressure parameters, let's get her down to radiology." That term, I knew, meant danger. Vasospasm—what we'd been hoping against hope wouldn't happen. After yet another CT scan, Dr. Johnson told us it was a critical time.

"She may die or suffer another stroke. Spend as much time with her as you can." He touched her on the foot and left the room. Fleeting appearance, swift disappearance. He had responded with calculated reservation and simply gave the information that he needed to convey. Now, I was left alone with my mother and my fears. I felt lost, unprepared. Helpless.

It was at that point the rage seeped in. This wasn't part of our plans. She was supposed to live. My parents were supposed to grow old together. Why her?

I left the hospital that day, darting across the atrium with my head down. I needed to be away from this place. The hospital was the embodiment of pain and frustration. Distance would help me clear my head, or at least get me to a place where I could sort through the web of thoughts.

As soon as I was in my car, I worried that something would happen to my mother while I was gone. The worst seemed inevitable, and I couldn't push away the fear of not being present if she were . . . to die. I felt powerlessness in the earthquake-like destruction that had crumbled her life and, by extension, my life. I felt indiscriminate rage at everything, at my own inability—impotence, actually—in fixing anything. There were no solutions, nothing for us to do by hunkering down as a family to resolve. Fixing my mother was completely out of my hands.

Everything was in Dr. Johnson's hands, in my mother's responses to the treatment, in her physical condition, in chance. All we could do was pray. We called in our family's Hindu priest, and he prayed with us at my mother's bedside, reciting mantras for us to repeat. It gave us something to do, it helped us find serenity. Our powerlessness was replaced with tranquility and hope, if only for a moment.

My mother's vasospasm increased.

Then it plateaued.

Then it fell on a downward slope.

I took a breath.

Ten days after her operation, two nurses came in while I sat with my mother to see if they could wash her hair, finally. For me, this was a project, and I was newly energized. I'd tried to comb it earlier, but the mats that had formed had grown too thick, and I worried about creating tension that would cause my mom any more pain or, worse, tear the new healing skin on the side of her head.

They set a pink wash basin against her neck and washed her head gently with baby shampoo. I took up the comb and tried again, but the teeth crunched into the matted hair, making things worse. My mom winced, then said, "That's okay." I tried again, to no avail.

The nurse stopped me. "We need to shave it. There is no other way."

Not my mother's hair.

"Oh dear," my mom said, and my heart broke. But then, she shrugged. "I guess . . . whatever you think is best."

My mom didn't have an opinion on this?

"It will grow back, Mom," I said, clearing my throat, trying to sound positive.

The nurse left and then returned with an electric razor. "Here," she said, holding it out to me. She didn't want to be the one to do it.

It seems like such a small thing in the abstract. It's only hair. But it was her hair. She had always taken such pride in grooming and curling her thick black hair that it was rarely out of place. And I had never shaved anybody's head before. I hadn't even trimmed anyone's hair. I had cut my dog's hair a few times, using the razor, but that was back when I was young. And it was my dog.

I hid the emotions before she could see my face. How bold and brave I'd always believed myself to be, but now, could I really say that I was a tiger? Was I anything more than a vulnerable cub? What I wanted was to collapse, for my mother—suddenly recovered—to stand up and tell me what to do. What would she have said?

"Sheri, just do it. Just take it off."

My mother needed me to be strong for her now. I took the razor, flipped the switch, felt the vibrations as it buzzed awake. I started in the front above her stapled incision and continued the work begun before surgery. I worked like a gardener might mow the lawn: a long stripe, front-to-back. Some of the hair fell away onto the pillow, some clung stubbornly to the matted lock. Front-to-back, another stripe. Then another. A larger chunk fell onto the white pillowcase. Fresh, pale scalp appeared across my mother's head, a waxing moon.

"Almost there, Mom."

She turned her head for me, and then I moved around the bed to the other side. The last of it fell onto the pillow, a halo of dark hair circling her head.

"How do I look?"

I dusted a lock off her forehead. "You look great, Mom. Just like a brand-new baby."

She laughed an uneasy laugh, but she was lucid enough to know that her hair was the least of her concerns at the moment.

The nurses collected the hair into a bag and disposed of it.

After two weeks in the intensive care unit, her vasospasm was on the continuous downward trajectory of the arterial ratios, which I'd learned meant that the spasm was slowly breaking. We could see that she was improving. Although confused and anxious at times, she seemed oriented. We dared to say it looked like she was going to survive this.

During that time I turned twenty-three. My two best friends from high school and my cousin brought a cake into my mother's room at the ICU. At first, I had balked, not interested in celebrating until my father said, "Sheri, this is important too. We want to celebrate this as a family." He was right. My mother wasn't quite sure what was going on and apologized to my friends for not cleaning up the house before the party. My friends were comforting and full of kind words. I could almost take a breath. Still, I was pretending to celebrate. I really just wanted to be left alone to focus on my mother.

Watching her that evening, I knew things weren't going to be the same. I worried about her career, how long it would be before she could get back to work. With her illness, I felt vulnerable, a bundle of exposed raw nerves. Here we were, eating cake as if it was all normal.

Four weeks after surgery, my mother's railroad scar glowed pink and scabbed, and Dr. Johnson began removing the small, white external catheter that had been draining my mom's spinal fluid into a bag. She was becoming untethered from the equipment that had been sustaining her. Dr. Johnson put in a small stitch where the catheter had been, and I marveled at the memory of having watched fluid drain into the bag for a month, how medieval it all was. However, as the day went on, a small trickle of white fluid appeared from the stitch, like a faucet with a slow drip. Then the drip wasn't so slow anymore. It widened, grew faster. It drained down the side of her eye. My mother had ordered a cup of coffee, and as I sat with her, occasionally trying to catch the drips with a towel, a few drips of fluid inched dangerously close to her mouth. I was horrified at the thought that it could get in the coffee. A couple of times, I caught it at the corner of her mouth before it dropped down to her gown and possibly into her cup. I gagged. The whole scene was disgusting. Whenever I was doing work back in the lab, if we had a cut or gash, we had to immediately cover it to avoid bacterial entrance. If my mother's stitch was leaking out, there was an opening, and, if she was wiping it away, I pictured all the bacteria, forming its masses, spreading throughout her body.

I asked the nurse if this was a major problem, or if there was something that we needed to do right now, and she paged Dr. Johnson.

It took a while for him to arrive, and I did what I could, semi-panicked, to keep my mother from touching (or accidentally drinking) the leaky fluid. When he did arrive, weary from surgery, but still positive, he told me he'd fix it right up and had me stand outside for a minute. "Alright, Dr. Dewan," he said to my mother, "just one stitch and then we're done."

I heard her say "ouch" in a voice gravelly and unfamiliar and not at all like my mother's, and then Dr. Johnson came out and said, "She's good to go. We'll get her to rehab as soon as possible." Then he shook my hand and was out the door, disappearing to some other part of the hospital. That was it. His work with my mom, and with me, was essentially complete.

I might have processed that with more lucidity in the moment, but the following day was my mother's fiftieth birthday. A day Jiji and I had planned on celebrating in big, Indian fashion, with her family and colleagues and friends, renting out a local banquet hall.

My dad, Jiji, and I got her a small cake, but my mother complained the whole time that her legs hurt. She halfheartedly chewed a piece of cake, which dried and crumbled in her parched mouth. All I could think was that my mother deserved better than this. The aneurysm didn't feel like a punishment, more like an injustice, or a terrible spin of the cosmic wheel.

Only later, and once my mother was in rehab, was I really able to start thinking again about the impact Dr. Johnson had on my mother's life, and especially on mine. I'd known about neurosurgeons, though I had never met one until my mother's illness. As a child, I'd thought about becoming a neurosurgeon in a sort of vague, fascinated way of someone who had lofty goals. Now, I was the very smart neuroscience student who could barely shave my mother's head. Who gagged at the sight of the spinal fluid leaking from a loose stitch. Who struggled to look at the stapled wound in my mother's head. Could I really be a neurosurgeon?

Yet, I had to wonder, was it the fluid, the scar, the staples that had bothered me most or the fact that all this was on my mother's head?

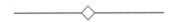

My mother would always be the one to say, "If you want to do it, then do it." She was ever a lover of a good anecdote, and more than once did she call up to Jiji and me (and did I overhear her relate to others) President Kennedy's moonshot speech. She was always quoting historical leaders, people who took up the mantle and said, "Yes, let's do this."

The title of Kennedy's moonshot speech, also known as "We Choose to Go to the Moon," was actually titled, "The Address at Rice University on the Nation's Space Effort." It was given on September 12, 1962, in the midst of the space race with the Soviet Union. The whole speech is worth reading (or watching), but the most famous portion is in the middle: "But why, some say, the moon? Why choose this as our goal? And they may well ask why climb the highest mountain? Why, thirty-five years ago, fly the Atlantic? Why does Rice play Texas? We choose to go to the moon. We choose to go to the moon in this decade and do the other things, not because they are easy, but because they are hard, because that goal will serve to organize and measure the best of our energies and skills, because the challenge is the one that we are willing to accept, one we are unwilling to postpone, and one which we intend to win . . . "[1]

There's no reason not to go for the big dream or the hard goal. Dreams are not the space to say I'm not good enough or smart enough or talented enough or rich enough or XYZ reasons or excuses.

However, it's also important to note that you might not be able to go to your door and begin your journey to your dream immediately. I wasn't ready to set off a few months after my mother's near-death experience, in the middle of her rehabilitation, and become a neurosurgeon right away. There was too much going on at home, too much in my life, too much grief I needed to process. Without processing that grief, I would have been creating chronic stress for myself, which is what we all need to avoid. But the seeds were planted, my origin story was forming, and I didn't let that dream die. I stayed on my adjacent path, not fully realizing at the time that I was laying the groundwork for my future.

2

Map It

In Kennedy's moonshot speech, he also related some of the details for how American astronauts would get to the moon, explaining that NASA would double the number of scientists and engineers, increasing salaries and expenses to $60 million a year, then spend $200 million on plant and laboratory facilities, build a rocket more than three hundred feet tall, with expert equipment for propulsion, guidance, control, communications, food and survival, and that it would all be done within the decade of the sixties.[1] What he was giving the audience at Rice, and indeed the world, was an explanation of how the moon landing would be achieved. Money was the first step. That money would be going toward the people who would have to then build all the different elements, which was why the space budget was so big.

When he gave this speech, the space program was already underway and while not all the particulars were yet known—the engineers would have to figure out the shapes of rockets, how to couple with the lander, and so forth—the engineers and the Kennedy administration understood what the process would entail for a successful moon landing. Kennedy's speech offered the public a layperson's map; meanwhile, NASA's engineers had their own very technical map. The dream of going to the moon was millennia old, the stuff of myth and legends around the world, but Jules Verne offered a fantastical (but logistical) approach in 1865, which became one of the first stories to be filmed in Georges Méliès' adaptation of the book in the 1902 silent film *A Trip to the Moon*. As soon as there were films, depictions of moon flight were a ready subject.

By the middle of the century, NASA had mapped the path to make the stuff of fiction a reality, once and for all.

The reason to focus on the moon is to show how achievable even the seemingly impossible can be. This requires steps, a plan, logistics, acquired knowledge, plenty of study and lots of perseverance. Despite all these hard tasks, humanity does this all the time.

What is more human than to set those big dreams and find a way to achieve them?

This is where grit alone isn't always helpful and certainly not a one-size-fits-all approach. You need to come up with your way forward that's personalized for your experience. Fortunately, mapping out a way to persevere and reach a goal can work for any goal, any dream, especially one that feels daunting at first.

The brain loves maps. It's like making an image for the brain to follow, a visualization of something that can be achieved. Visualization triggers your occipital lobe, which is where you can "see" what you're thinking. This also activates the brain's frontal lobe, which is the part of your brain you use for learning, planning, and then executing the plans. Replaying these visualizations in your mind orients your pesky fight-or-flight amygdala responses. Essentially, your fears are adapting to your vision. The obvious benefit is that this acclimation lowers anxiety around that particular goal. When you truly visualize an action, your brain stimulates your motor pathways to your muscles, as if you're actually going through the motions already, habituating your brain and body to the act itself. Athletes and musicians will especially recognize this phenomenon.

Here's the thing: you want to have a detailed plan, but it's also important to understand that things may not go according to your perfectly set out plan. You may need to change strategies, narrow the focus, make the occasional detour, or even modify part of your goal. Most of the time, your path won't be linear. The key is not to get derailed. Your brain can adapt to this new information; that's the beauty of its structure. While our brain is designed to recognize patterns (following instructions), the brain also has a great capacity to grow and change and evolve—that's neuroplasticity. We use neuroplasticity every day to connect and reorganize neural networks. This allows us to learn from failures and "rewire" using alternate strategies.

Dr. Doug Johnson's ability to save my mother's life inspired me; I felt in my heart that was what I wanted to do. However, I was a student and had a mother with neurologic trauma. How could I simply embark on a new, very difficult, and demanding course of study?

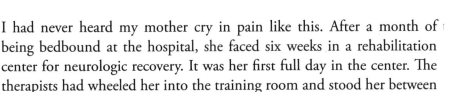

I had never heard my mother cry in pain like this. After a month of being bedbound at the hospital, she faced six weeks in a rehabilitation center for neurologic recovery. It was her first full day in the center. The therapists had wheeled her into the training room and stood her between two parallel bars to brace herself while she practiced walking again. Her severely atrophied legs collapsed under the weight.

"My legs hurt," she said, over and over, wailing with each step. The soft peach fuzz of her new-growth hair stood out all over her scalp, around the puckered pink scar. I thought of an old railroad overgrown with dandelions.

"Come on, Mrs. Dewan, I know it hurts, but we have to build those muscles back up for you. The more we get you up and walking around, the sooner they'll stop hurting."

I watched from inside the family viewing area off to the side, designed to stop our temptation of helping too much. There was absolutely nothing I could do for her. If I was a tiger, all I could do was roar; but from inside a cage, with no one around to listen, I was a mewling cub.

A couple of times, I had to turn away as my mother collapsed and the therapist got her back up. Her surgical ordeal was over, and while I knew rehab would be work, I expected my mother to be able to tackle this like any other task she had undertaken. When we hiked through the Himalayas, I couldn't even remember her complaining about a blister, let alone crying that something hurt. Who was this woman, crying, emotional, distracted, and wanting to give up?

I called over to her, "Mom, it's just a few more steps. You can do this."

My mother shook her head.

"Mrs. Dewan, we just need you to do a little bit more. Then, I promise, you can lie back down in bed, and we'll do other activities with you."

"Actually," I said, "she's Doctor Dewan. She has a PhD." I didn't know why it bothered me to hear her called *Mrs.* instead of *Dr.* Of course, I couldn't articulate it at the time, but what I needed was some reminder of my mother's dignity. Her old self. The person I couldn't see at all in that rehabilitation center.

"Oh, I'm sorry," the therapist said. "Dr. Dewan, you can take five more steps for me, can't you?"

She made it through the steps, and then the therapist wheeled her back to her room, where I rubbed her legs, pressing the muscles to give her relief. We did this for her every day, alternating between me, Jiji, and my dad, warming the cream in our hands then working the knots of her muscles on her thin, withered legs.

The therapists were kind, but beyond that, the rehab center appeared a house of suffering. The inpatients endured a variety of neurologic disorders, including strokes, paralysis, and traumatic brain injury. There were craniotomy scars of every size, shape, and color, all in various stages of healing. Some scars were on the front of the head, some in the back, some on the side, some still with staples, some with black or blue sutures.

After a week there, my mom told me that some of the patients frightened her. Though they were in a lockdown unit, they were loud at night, rowdy, and the aggressive sounds from within echoed through the otherwise quiet halls. Some of the patients were "frontal," exhibiting a loss of inhibitions and self-control. When it was time for me to say goodnight, my mother held my wrist. "I don't want to be alone. It's scary." We couldn't stay overnight with her, though. She had only been there for one week, but she was terrified to be alone at night. I wasn't sure if she could take five more weeks at the rehab center.

When it came time for the next meeting with my mother's case manager, I sat in her cramped office, expecting a regular rundown of my mother's progress, ready to suggest we bring my mother home. Then the case manager turned toward me, "So what are the next steps for your mother?"

"Well, she's of course going to go back to work," I said. "She's a professor. Ideally, I think she'd like to be back for the fall semester."

The case manager looked at me, not unkindly, and said in a no-nonsense voice, "Um, you need to fill out disability paperwork for her."

"Disability? What are you talking about? She doesn't have a disability." Who was this person trying to tell me that my mother had a disability? Didn't she have any sense of who my mother was?

"I know it's a stressful time and paperwork is the last thing you want to deal with, but the reality is that your mother has suffered severe neurologic trauma. It's always good to stay positive, but you still need to prepare for the likelihood that she won't return to the way she was. It's likely, especially with older stroke patients, that she may never work again."

Older? My mom wasn't older, she was only fifty. I stared her down. Who was she to tell me that my mom wouldn't work again? According to her job title, she was not a doctor. The case manager was seeing only this carcass of my mother's normal self. "My mom is a smart, educated, talented woman. She doesn't just sit around. This is only temporary."

"Of course, she *was* all those things." Her voice was stern, and the way she emphasized "was" set me off. I could tell she was growing impatient, but that was fine by me. "But she is not all these things right now. And you really need to fill out this paperwork for the state."

Nope. No way, lady. "You don't seem to understand. You don't make decisions for my mother's life without her, and I'm not about to take away her career when she's too sick to do anything about it."

"I'm sorry," she said, her lips pursed, "but your mother is unable to make these decisions. As her family, you now have to make these critical choices for her. This is part of being a caretaker. She needs to have this done for her if she's going to go back to work.

"Your mother has had a stroke. That will affect her cognition for a long time, perhaps forever. We will work very hard for her recovery, but you have to accept that things may never be the same again. You must prepare for that."

She slid the documents over to my side of the desk. I took a cursory look but made sure to show all the disdain I felt. Then I said, "I'm sure you think you know patients, but you don't know my mother. She is not disabled. She had an aneurysm, it was fixed. There was a stroke, but she's going to recover. The fog will lift, and she *will* go back to work." I was digging my foxhole of stubborn hubris and family pride. And denial.

The case manager shook her head. "I'm sure she will recover, but recovery looks different for all patients. Recovery means functioning, but it doesn't always mean 100 percent. What I'm saying is that you can't neglect your duties to your mother. This is important paperwork, and you need to take into account her current condition. You'll need to prepare yourself in case she is unable to go back to work." She picked up the packet and held it out for me to take. "And I do see many, many patients. I go through this every day. This is the paperwork you need to fill out. This isn't for my benefit. This is for your mother's. For your family's." Her annoyance matched mine, but this paper pusher was not about to tell me what my family did or didn't need.

"I'm not signing a thing." I stood up and stormed out of the office.

I was a twenty-three-year-old telling a middle-aged professional her job and refusing to acknowledge that it was possible my mom would not be the way she was before her illness. It had never once occurred to me that this wasn't just a blip. My mother didn't die in the hospital. Okay, that was an illness, and she was no longer ill; we were just working to get back to the old life. We'd one day look back on all of this and give a sigh of relief, feeling pleased with ourselves for overcoming a struggle together.

That meeting was not my finest moment. While the case manager might not have had the best bedside manner either, she was giving me a dose of truth, which was the last thing I wanted to hear.

I told my father about the exchange as soon as I got home. He was surprised when I mentioned the disability paperwork, but he didn't share my anger. "Now, what did she say?" he asked.

"That I had to be realistic, and that she probably would never work again."

My father shook his head. "That doesn't sound like your mother."

"Exactly. That's what I said."

"What would she do if she couldn't work again?"

"It just wouldn't happen. I told her that she didn't know my mother."

After a moment's reflection, he said, "But don't you think it's wise to fill out the paperwork?"

I hoped my father wasn't about to side with the case manager. "Why would we do that to Mom? We would be making a decision for her future without her say-so. We can't do that. We can't take away her career!"

"I agree. But if she has to take off work for a longer period of time, maybe there's a way to apply for temporary disability."

I grumbled, but I liked the word temporary. I could deal with temporary.

"And remember that the case manager is only trying to help," my father said. "It might be good to listen to what she has to say. And then she can eat her words when your mother exceeds everyone's expectations. But for now, we must be accepting of recommendations."

That night, my brain wouldn't shut off. I was still angry, and I made it my mission to direct my anger toward the case manager. Temporary.

That's all this was—wasn't it? But that insidious word. Disability. The permanence of it. People *became* disabled, and that was their new state. People recovered from strokes, though. People even went back to work after strokes. Okay, maybe they weren't exactly the same.

And then I thought of my mother, unable to remember words, her struggle to walk. And then there were the other patients in the rehab center; the stroke patients were struggling. Their families were struggling. How naïve were my expectations of a perfect recovery, a total erasure of the illness? I wasn't ready to acknowledge that the case worker had a point, or that my mother was in fact disabled, or that I had been rude, or that I was not coping as well as I thought, or that I might spend the rest of my mother's life being her caretaker. But there it all was, plenty of rational facts laid out in front of me: the seriousness of my mother's condition, the very slow recovery she had ahead, the shrinking likelihood that she would be ready to teach in a few months' time.

All of this made my next visit to the rehab center worse. My mother was a part of this house of horrors. Everyone in here was somebody's loved one, and now they all were neurologically impaired and could possibly be impaired forever. Even my mother.

Still in denial, we managed to convince the director that we could take care of my mother at home and bring her in for the necessary outpatient therapies (after much insistence to combat the director's skepticism).

"We're a close family. We've always taken care of each other. This is just one more challenge we can face." It sounded like a speech from a cheesy '80s movie about teens on a school trip getting stranded on an island.

We were adamant, though. Our biggest argument was that she would recover better at home, surrounded by familiarity, where she wasn't terrified. Finally, the director signed the paperwork, and within that week, we brought my mother back home. At least, we brought back the woman who had been my mother.

My father and I drove her home and helped her out of the car. We brought her into the house. She looked around, almost dazed.

"You are home, dear," my father said. My mother didn't react.

We took her through every room, and she looked at all of her things, a little confused. The rooms might have been vaguely familiar; it was almost as if she was looking at it through a lens of a faded memory: Oh, these are my clothes. These are my shoes. This is my life. Okay.

I couldn't tell if it meant anything to her; she showed no emotions.

The woman we brought home was a changeling mother. Or, at least, she was the surviving shell that retained only a fraction of my mother. This mother was quiet. She was docile and pensive. On top of that, the woman who always had a book in her hand was unable to read and couldn't concentrate for more than a few minutes. She would sit for extended periods on the couch and complain of her head. Her conversations were brief, interrupted by episodes of confusion. She quickly forgot names, dates, and times, and sometimes even people, which stressed her out. Dr. Johnson had made her body whole, but her mind was in a faraway place, searching through dense fog to return home.

Her mind had been stolen. I told myself it didn't matter that she wasn't exactly the same. She was alive. She would get better each day. She had to.

On her second day home, I gave her a bath. Just like you would do with a baby, I filled the tub, checked the temperature, then lowered my mom into the bathwater. I shampooed the layer of hair that was ever so slightly growing back, and I was careful to put only light pressure on her scar. Then, I tilted back her head and rinsed out the soap. Next, I scrubbed her down with a sponge, gentle on the skin that seemed as delicate as the parchment paper my mother had used for baking. I poured water over her shoulders, down her back. I washed every part of my mother. I wanted to cry the whole time, but I did my best to push it down.

"That's nice. Thank you, Sheri," she said in a flat voice. "I think I can do this myself next time."

She was right. I sat with her for her next bath, and she did just fine.

It was just that I could never leave her alone.

I learned there were certain tasks she could do with relative ease, the rote mechanics of movement that were embedded into her motor cortex. A few days after coming home, my mom wanted to make herself a cup of tea. She loved tea, had usually made some for herself every day. So, I watched her as she filled the kettle, put the kettle on the burner, then started the burner. All of these methodical, rote activities that she did without a thought. Then, she removed a cup from the cabinet, poured a spoon of sugar into the cup, got the tea bag, and put it into the empty cup. I was so relieved. *Ha, and the director didn't think she could handle things at home!* I was thrilled with her progress in such a short time.

Except . . . my mom left the kitchen. She went into the living room, looked at the spines of the books on the bookshelves, and sat down on her chair, picking up a magazine. The kettle started to whistle. My mom didn't react. *Okay,* I thought, *it's taking time to process, that's all.*

Ten seconds.

Twenty seconds.

The kettle's whistling increased. My mother looked at something on the couch, maybe a piece of lint. She flipped through the magazine.

Thirty seconds.

Forty seconds.

"Mom!" I said. "I think your tea water is ready!"

"Oh! I had forgotten all about it."

I brought her home from therapy one day to an awful smell in the house, only to realize that five days earlier, my mom had attempted to do laundry and left the clothes in the washer to mold. And, somehow, we'd all missed it. We were exhausted. This was the kind of low I had never known before. The fear of my mother's death had been there, and strong, but this, this was weeks of fatigue and anguish. I think we were all a little depressed in dealing with this new way of life, for my mom and for us all. There was no One Terrible Thing, just the exhausting grind of making sure my mother didn't burn down the house . . . or hurt herself . . . or break something. Plus—there was still the fear of death. Mine and Jiji's.

Ever since Dr. Johnson had recommended Jiji and I have an MRA (magnetic resonance angiography) because aneurysms could be hereditary, I could picture in my brain a tiny, ballooning artery swelling against brain tissue that could explode at any time and alter my life forever. Or end it.

Between chasing my mother around the house and administering to her every need, I read different books on aneurysms or searched the internet for statistics. They're more common in women who smoke. My mother never smoked a cigarette in her life. Aneurysms are more common in women with high blood pressure. I wouldn't say her blood pressure was high, but my mother did have a Type A personality. She was always racing from one task to another. Was that cause or coincidence? Was it hereditary? If so, I would get the test, but I couldn't deal with that now. Once things were back on track with my mom, then yes, I'd get it done.

Still, looking at my mother forced me into dark places, imagining myself in the hospital, head shaved, a scar down the side of my scalp, turning on burners, leaving tasks half-finished, unable to process reading, losing everything I had. There were days when, "This could be me," morphed into, "This will be me." I would show up to my lab convinced that I was about to save the world and all of humanity, only to return home and feel a deep hopelessness. My mom wasn't going to get better. I probably had an aneurysm that would burst in my head at any time.

All of this emotional fluctuation made me irritable, short-fused, especially when my mother asked repetitive questions, or couldn't remember something I had just said, or wandered out of the room after putting a pot of pasta on the stove or leaving milk on the counter or couldn't say words clearly. I felt trapped, angry at things beyond anyone's control.

In that time, my father stepped into what had been her role. Not only did he still have to go to work, but he now also took care of the household in every aspect, at least when Jiji and I weren't around to help. My father had built up enough seniority in a job that had always been consistently 8:00 a.m. to 5:00 p.m. that he had flexibility to take some time off, or he would arrange to have my mother cared for during the day. Jiji and I struggled in our own way. It was our mother who had been our rock, our center.

My mother's neurologist recommended putting her on mood-stabilizing medication, and at first, I was resistant to the idea of more medications.

"Well," the neurologist said, "strokes are different entities. Strokes can change the brain. These would be mood-stabilizing medications, and they would be temporary."

Temporary lit up like a giant neon sign. *Temporary* was the word I wanted to hear, what made everything seem a little bit better. The neurologist explained MAOI inhibitors—the serotonin uptake pills that would keep her on a more even keel and, most importantly, that she wouldn't need forever. I clung to that with the faintest flicker of hope.

My inner tiger also felt sheepish about my behavior with the case manager at the rehab center. I was falling apart and wanted someone to blame for the upheaval in my family. I wanted to have all the answers to be strong for my mother, but I felt like I was failing her. I also had it in my head that signing the paperwork was akin to failure of her dreams, as if ending her career earlier than intended negated all the work she had accomplished. On top of that, I was ashamed that, after all my mom tried to teach me, I had behaved immaturely and was out of control. With no one in my family to really discuss this with, and no desire to dwell on my behavior and the enumeration of my fears, I did my best to push that all out of my mind and view my mother's recovery as a series of tasks to undertake. Put away as many emotions as I could.

My dad tried to find humor in her paraphasic errors (the misuse or substitution of words); my mom even laughed at herself sometimes. Other times, she'd forget a friend's name when they came to visit, or she couldn't remember the friend at all. Then came the "why me" phase, and she spent days staring into space at nothing.

But I did begin to see sparks. There were subtle, gradual improvements in my mother. She would read a paragraph and remember small details. She complained less about the pain in her head. There were clear daily goals for her to follow as her brain relearned how to map out a day. Routine . . . ritual . . . therapies.

Names came more easily to her, and she could hold onto thoughts a little longer. As her brain healed, the fog slowly began to clear. The tea was poured into cups. Laundry was moved to the dryer and then folded. Nothing burned down, not even a singe. My mental map for my mom was to get her back to her pre-aneurysm self, and though I needed to learn for myself what my mom's new goal could be, the therapists and doctors had given us a map of achievable milestones to use as a guide. Once we had a map, we found a way to help get her there.

As her brain healed, I relaxed, and my stress lessened. My inner tiger didn't feel quite so caged. I could contemplate my own next steps and get back to mapping my path to a clear goal. What was I going to do with my life now? My mother's illness had been a break, but it also made room for a pause, for a chance to reflect.

First, I needed to find a job. Since research had been a part of my biology undergraduate training, I found an in vitro fertilization lab close to my parents' house that needed technicians to run assays for patients who were getting hormones tested to aid with pregnancy. The lab was easily drivable, so I sent in an application. Within a few days, I was hired.

The pay was seventeen dollars an hour. I had never made money like that before; it was a financial windfall of pocket money, as far as I was concerned. And the assays that I was performing were changing the lives of patients. I didn't always get to see the patients, but sometimes I would be around when they dropped off their samples at the lab, and I would interact with them briefly to receive the vials. They were all women desperate to conceive. The work wasn't really about anonymous tubes of blood—they were real women.

I had the short-term covered: job, duties at home, mom's recovery. I had money coming in, I enjoyed the work, and I had peace of mind. Allowing myself the space and time to focus on doing only the things that absolutely needed to get done, I got to a place with more clarity, more room for taking on new tasks. As my mother healed, so did I.

What I needed was to figure out my new plan. My mother's aneurysm had disrupted all of our plans and had shaken our family to its very core. Once again, I latched on to the word *temporary*. I would not be my mother's caretaker and companion forever. I certainly had no intentions of running assays as a lab technician forever, though it was an excellent job. But I had always intended it to be the bridge to what came next. It was time to start that next phase.

I wanted to find a way to return someone's mother to them someday, to be capable of adding more time to someone's life. I could do this with my research, by studying aneurysms and strokes and Alzheimer's, both prevention and cures. Research was what I knew and what I loved. Researchers could make advancements in the way that neurosurgeons treat patients. Or maybe . . . I could do even more immediate work. What was stopping me from being more than a researcher?

Surgery had saved my mother's life; I could make an impact as a neurosurgeon. I could be Dr. Johnson, not the bowtie, but the scrubs, the confidence, the cutting into someone's brain, and placing a lifesaving metal clip on an aneurysm. There was the image of neurosurgery ahead of me, I could almost see it, see myself in the operating room, but now that it was time to think about heading down that road, I had too many doubts.

A year ago, my mom had told me that if I wanted something badly enough, there was nothing that could stop me. I might not get it right away, but I could plan in the meantime.

Everyone knows neurosurgery is one of the toughest pursuits, requiring an inhumanly rigorous course of study and an uncommon sense of hubris. But now all my reserves were depleted. I did not have the energy, the resilience, or the fortitude for that kind of undertaking just yet. I needed more time.

Instead, I applied to a graduate program in neuroscience. Northwestern University had a master's program that included research as well as neuroscience coursework. I still wasn't sure if I was better suited for research or medicine, but this program would give me the opportunity to discover where I should be. My acceptance to the master's program was the spark of good news that my family needed at the time. My mother told me she was happy for me, that she was proud of me, albeit with a lethargic smile. It was a relief that I would be staying close to home and, from the lab on the Evanston Campus at Northwestern, could go back and forth at a moment's notice in case of an emergency.

I felt a new charge, as though I was taking control over my life after having been forced into the backseat, helplessly watching trauma unfold while lacking knowledge or skills to make an impact. Before I could blink, I was four months into my master's coursework in neuroscience, and I was all in with my research, fascinated with everything I was discovering.

I set out a map, one I knew could fork to two different paths, but still, I was able to have a tangible goal and make the steps. It's hard to say whether it was a total detour, but if I did become a neurosurgeon, it would only help that I already knew so much about the brain.

And not all detours are bad. As it turns out, aside from making lifelong friends during this time, I met my husband, Alex, who was a biochemistry PhD candidate.

Alex had lost his mother to a rare disease, so he understood the space I needed to continue to heal, and we offered each other mutual support. It was when he took me home to first meet his dad and cadre of aunts and grandmothers—all professional women and tigers in their own right— and they discussed future options with me that I realized I was, at last, ready to think seriously about medicine.

I was at the fork in my path. To the left, I could enter a life as a PhD scientist and researcher, devoting my days to the lab, writing grants, conducting experiments, and becoming truly academic. To the right, there was life as a medical doctor, a surgeon, potentially a neurosurgeon. Both doors opened onto very lengthy paths with somewhat uncertain futures.

Neurosurgery was a tantalizing proposition. It was the apex of medical science and pinnacle of difficulty. I was the diligent worker, but it was always Jiji who had been the brilliant student. Would my skills and work ethic, my intelligence, really be enough to do the work? I wanted to do the hardest thing, but I also had a dream when I was young to climb Mount

Everest, and I knew that was far beyond my skill level. (I had to be satisfied with seeing it from afar, when my mom and I took our trip through the Annapurna range, which was a difficult enough trek.)

The few times I had ventured to share my interest in neurosurgery outside of my family, I was met with surprise and derision. Neurosurgery wasn't something young women did. Normally, this would have steeled my resolve to pursue it, but I knew, too, that the path to becoming a neurosurgeon was grueling. Patients would live and die under my hand. I wouldn't have regular hours or a regular life, and here I was, now with the person I imagined I'd spend the rest of my life with. Would that be fair to him? There were many reasons why neurosurgery was an inspiring but unlikely dream. And besides, it wasn't as if I was being a slouch by choosing neuroscience research.

Deep down, I had known years earlier that I wanted to be a doctor. And the more I had time to reflect, the more I knew I wanted to be in an operating room over a research lab. Once I'd had nearly two years to take a breath, let the stress of my mother's illness and recovery release, and watch her actually improve, my need to be challenged reasserted itself. Of course, I wanted to do the hardest thing possible. Alex, too, reassured me he would support whatever dream I wanted to follow.

My next concrete step on my path: medical school. Maybe there I'd find the certainty in my direction I'd been seeking all these years. So, once I finished my master's program, I applied to medical school and was admitted for the fall.

———————◇———————

Make a path. Write it down. Visualize. Let the brain get accustomed to seeing it play out so the goal becomes real, tangible, a focal point—the idea has moved from a series of processes between neurons and into something that can be seen on a page. When I was a kid, I made a list of all the places I wanted to see when I grew up, chronicled them as a promise to myself, and eventually the older I got, the more I was (and continue to be) able to check those places off my list. As silly or simplistic as it may seem, writing down *any* type of goal—a daily to-do list, a list of requirements for graduation, a step-by-step outline of what it would take to become a neurosurgeon, a list of exercises for occupational therapy to be able to walk and use your hands and complete daily functions around the home—can concretize the goal. The brain knows it's now accountable to that list—which is important if it really is your moonshot.

3

Don't Take Surveys

Consulting experts is frequently a good approach when needing to learn more about a particular field or making a decision. Likewise, talking with people who support you can be comforting and help give you clarity on what direction to take.

However . . .

Be wary of taking surveys. Of consulting with everyone who has an opinion. Even, at times, the purported experts. Let me explain.

I mentioned earlier that when I'd talk about my dream of becoming a neurosurgeon, I was met with surprise and derision. Even a stubborn and driven person like me was nearly derailed from following my dream because of these naysayers. This doesn't mean that feedback is never good, but if you find yourself asking everyone the "Should I?" questions, consider that you might be stalling on purpose or second-guessing yourself.

I've had naysayers both as the expert as well as the armchair-expert variety. Much of the naysaying came unsolicited, so be prepared to ignore a lot of people—they're white noise, and they have a myriad of reasons for their own feelings, 99 percent of which don't involve you at all.

———————◇———————

When I was still an undergraduate, before my mother's illness, my family and I attended an outdoor picnic with members of the local Indian community. It was their annual summer party, attended by the usual acquaintances, friends, and plenty of people we didn't know. Some of these people worked with my mother on taking students back to India for her study trips, so largely, it was a networking event and a chance to speak Hindi and eat great food. I took this as a chance to get excited for the upcoming trip my mother and I had planned in the summer. We would be going to India to see my grandmother, perhaps one last time, and then hike through the Annapurnas. I was ecstatic.

While I delved into the *dham*, I struck up a conversation with an elderly family friend. We sat down together on a bench, out of the way of the children who were playing catch, the wheelbarrow race, and other makeshift games and contests.

"So," he said, "your mother tells me you will be finishing college soon."

"I have another year to go."

"Good, good. What are your interests? What do you think you'll do next?"

Though I still had plenty of questions for myself, I loved the chance to talk about my plans out loud to other people, not because I necessarily cared about their opinions—though to a certain extent I did—but because the more I talked about my plans, the more real and the more possible they seemed. This was part of my way of mapping my goal.

"I am actually fascinated with neuroscience," I told him in all eagerness. "I'm trying to decide whether I want to go to graduate school to become a researcher or go to medical school and become a neurosurgeon." Even then, the summer before my mother's aneurysm, before meeting Dr. Johnson, neurosurgery was at least on my mind as more than a childhood dream.

He sat back, slapped his hands on his thighs. "No, no, child. You shouldn't go into something like surgery. That's not for you. It's not for women."

I balked.

"No, child," he said, seeing my face, "you can be a doctor, but go into radiology. That way, you could still have a life, a family. It will be much easier for you to do it that way."

"But I'm not interested in radiology," I countered.

"You may not be as fulfilled with the job, but in the end, what's more important: your passion for your work or your family?"

There were plenty of things I wanted to say back to him, but I retracted my tiger claws and refrained. I reminded myself that he was from a different generation. I also reminded myself that what I did wasn't up to him, even if he dismissed my desires. This man certainly didn't know me better than I knew myself. I was annoyed, even a little angry. He never would have told a young man he couldn't be both a surgeon and a husband, a father.

Later on, I told my mother about what he said.

She listened, and then waved her hand once, as if swatting the story away. "If you want to be a neurosurgeon, you go ahead and do it." It was an authoritative declaration. That was all she said. All she had to say. She was a headstrong woman. I would be every bit as headstrong when it came to following my own path then, but I was fortunate to have a mother who would support me unconditionally . . . for as long as she was able.

I realize that not everyone has a supportive network within their families, which makes it all the more important to uphold your convictions.

The second naysayer was a little more shocking. That undergraduate summer of the picnic, I was also assisting a professor on his research project at Northwestern University's downtown campus. Every day, I took the train from my parents' house, where I was living during the summer, which dropped me off at the metro station downtown, where I picked up the Pace bus to the Northwestern Campus to get to the lab, then took the bus and the train back home—an hour and a half each way. (That's how badly I wanted this life; I knew it was an important step on my map to a career in either the medical or scientific field.) The professor was a PhD researcher who hadn't pursued the MD road. One day over lunch, he asked me, "What do you want to do with your life?"

Surgeon, I thought, even though at that point I was still toying with following the research path. Then neurosurgery flashed into my head. "I've always wanted to be a doctor and go to medical school."

He nodded. "Well, what do you ultimately want to achieve with that?" I respected the question, that he wanted to tease out how mapped out my path was.

I didn't have to think of my answer. "I know it sounds trite, but I want to help people. Someday, I want to do global-international charity work. I want to make a difference in people's lives, including people who don't have access to care." I'd learned enough from my mother to know how essential this was. I'd been brought up to see the disparities of global health and was told that I had the ability to do something to help, whatever path I chose.

Then, the professor's posture shifted, and he said, "That's very noble of you. But I wonder if you'll change your mind."

"What? Why?"

"Well," he said, "after you've done four years of medical school, a lengthy residency—depending on what you do—and then have all your medical school loans, have your patient practice, and have a life, are you really going to want to pick up and go to a different country to operate and do international work?" He laughed to himself, then repeated, "I just wonder if you'll change your mind."

He continued eating his salad with a smirk, as if he had just dispelled some great wisdom while taking delight in bursting some college student's dream. If he hadn't been so smug and condescending, I would have taken it more as cautionary advice, or maybe even the words of a cynic. Instead, I said, "I think I know myself, and I've grown up in a family dedicated to service," and left it at that. He was going to be on an already growing list of naysayers and detractors I was determined to prove wrong. It was one thing to be discouraged by older, traditional Indian men or researchers who didn't go into the medical field; it was quite another to hear it from the surgeons who are training you and your medical school colleagues. As I entered medical school, even among like-minded peers and actual doctors teaching us, there were still a few encounters with people who were more than eager to weigh negatively on my dreams.

The beginning of medical school is the study of Gross Anatomy, much of which is spent in learning overly complicated Greek- and Latin-based terminology such as *sphenopalatine ganglioneuralgia* and *diaphragmatic flutter*, which are the scientific terms for an ice cream headache and a hiccup, respectively. This was the first real academic struggle I ever had. For the first time, I had to study night and day, harder than I'd ever had before, making graduate school by comparison seem quaint and bucolic (incidentally, from the ancient Greek *boukolikón*, or cowherd). For a while, I worried I might have *iatromisia*, an aversion to medical practice, with a particular distaste for medical terms that are specifically Greek and Latin.

Year two of medical school is Physiology, Pathology, and Pharmacology. Medical students are still in the classrooms and labs, learning everything we can about the human body before actually treating patients.

The third and fourth years are spent in rotation, when medical students get their short, white coats and head to the hospitals. For eight weeks at a time, my classmates and I were assigned a hospital and a specialty somewhere in the metro Chicago area. (I spent a lot of time in the car those two years.) The obvious reason for this is to have a general understanding of all specialties; the *real* reason for rotations is to identify where in the medical field you fit in. By the end of that year, we would have to make official our specialty; we would have to choose what we were going to do for the rest of our lives based on a few weeks. Fortunately for me, I was sure my future lay in surgery. It's just that, while I felt the pull toward neurosurgery, I still had doubts as to whether I could, or should, pursue that field. The good news for me: one of the sub-internship rotations would be in neurosurgery.

It's critical for emergency room doctors to know a little bit about everything, and it's useful for every doctor to know how to deliver a baby. Every doctor should know the delicate and specific differences between treating children and adults. We all need to know how to recognize a heart attack, stroke . . . or aneurysm. Those could happen anywhere, anytime. (Yes, I was once, years later, on a plane when flight attendants made the call *Is there a doctor on board?* The situation turned out to be not that dramatic or involved, but I was able to help.)

My rotations began with an OB-GYN specialty at a hospital on the west side of Chicago, the kind of place where security had to walk us to our cars every night (my very first birth was assisting in a C-section to a fifteen-year-old girl, and most of the other thirteen babies were also to girls in their early- to mid-teens). I also worked in the clinic and saw so many young people with STDs, which was enough to make even the most stalwart stomach a little queasy.

At the end of this rotation, one of the women residents asked me what specialty I was thinking of pursuing. "Being an OB-GYN is really a great career," she said.

"I can see that," I said, having marveled at the awesome power of being present at the first breath of a tiny human. "But I'm," and there I paused, only because I was saying it now, out loud, to a stranger, now that I was officially on this path, "I think I'm leaning toward neurosurgery."

She looked at me askance, then blurted, "But—you're too pretty to be a neurosurgeon!"

Huh? I had no idea how to take that statement. It was the strangest and most off-putting, backhanded compliment I had ever received. Did neurosurgeons have reputations for being ogres? Was it a way of saying that I didn't look *smart enough* to be a neurosurgeon? Or that women doctors didn't really need lofty goals? "Uh, I—"

The resident read the awkwardness of the situation, then added, "It's just that—you're pretty. You don't need to do neurosurgery."

"Uh-huh. Thanks for the advice." I walked away.

I wasn't sure where that comment came from. Granted, I had already learned that residents (those undergoing their final in-hospital training for at least five years) were overworked and completely jaded, especially at a hospital that wasn't on, say, the north side of Chicago, with affluent patients and fewer emergencies and almost no lack of privilege. The residents here, and later on the south side, encountered a daily buffet of horrors without having enough doctors and staff to spread out said horrors. So, on that front, I sympathized and had a modicum of patience with a doctor who might say something uncouth, but I did feel different toward that OB-GYN resident after that encounter.

Yet, something in her comment triggered an impulse of defiance in me. Who was she to set the terms of my life? She was no gatekeeper of neurosurgery. It frustrated me endlessly that a woman couldn't be supportive of another woman's plan.

Even though I tried to move on with my day, I kept coming back to the OB-GYN's presumptuousness. By the end of my shift, annoyance escalated to anger, and though I wasn't outright rude to her, I didn't extend any niceties with her at all. It was bad enough having old men as detractors to becoming a neurosurgeon, but hearing it from a relatively young woman was akin to betrayal.

I went directly from OB-GYN on the west side to the ER rotation at Cook County Hospital, where the emergency room was regularly filled with the clamor of about two hundred patients, many of whom were lower income as well as indigent and overall desperate people. The body heat regularly kept the room at what felt like eighty degrees. After a few weeks of the ER rotation, I had my Pediatric rotation, also at Cook County Hospital, where I understood the full ramifications of childhood poverty in the United States.

Several months later, I *finally* got to my first surgical rotation where the burnout and cynicism were as rampant as ever. Many of us medical students were getting excited as we moved through our rotations because, at least for most of us, we were circling closer to selecting our specialty. At the end of this year, we would make our official decision with the office of the Dean of Medical Affairs. I had a good idea of what I was going to do, and my upcoming two-week neurosurgical rotation would help me know for sure. I felt fortunate that I had this pull early on. There were a few of my colleagues who still had no idea what they were going to do. Many agonized over their decisions. I realized I wasn't the only one with doubts, but at least I had *some* idea. More than half of our group leaned toward surgery.

My cohort, Roger, and I were discussing it one morning while waiting for our list of assignments. "I really want to be an orthopedic surgeon," he said.

"That's great. Why?" I asked. I was curious about what motivated my friends and colleagues toward their fields, always wondering what drove each of us to this moment.

"I don't know, I think it would be really cool. It's exciting, you know? You'd get to be in the operating room every day—" he stopped short. "But I really hate the operating room."

I tried to unpack what Roger had said. "How are you going to be an orthopedic surgeon if you don't like to be in the operating room?" It was exciting because he could be in a place he hated? That logic didn't make sense. And he didn't give an answer. He circled back to orthopedic surgeons being cool. I think he was enthralled by the mystique of being a surgeon but didn't want to deal with the day-to-day of it.

"What about you?" he asked.

"I'm—I'm really excited about neurosurgery."

He gave me a funny look. "Really? But those guys"—and I noted his use of guys— "they're so tough they drink their own pee!"

I cocked my head. *And I'm not tough?*

This was a line I'd heard before, and I was confident I knew from which surgical residents he'd cribbed it. Roger was a good guy, but still, I was frustrated that I only encountered negativity about becoming a neurosurgeon from nearly everyone I spoke with.

A couple of days later, when asked by one of the surgical residents what my preference was and I told her neurosurgery, she told me, in a very concerned voice, that if I became a neurosurgeon, my husband would leave me, and (with great emphasis) that I would never be able to have kids. Was there some memo somewhere that I hadn't read, setting out these very explicit rules?

Alex was my regular go-to for unloading all the varied hospital stories of the day, as the biological aspects intrigued him, but also, I was lucky he took a keen interest in what I was doing. As I was letting off steam that night about yet another colleague discrediting my dream, how so many people seemed to get in a tizzy because I wanted to be a neurosurgeon, he said, "Well, you know, neurosurgery's not exactly feminine."

Uh, what?

Was I really being naïve in thinking that I should pursue what I was interested in? "Does that mean I can't be a girl and do surgery?" I said with more than a little glibness.

"No, no, that's not it at all. I guess it just means . . . that you drill holes in people's heads. It's cool. But kinda. . .macho."

Now I was shocked. Despite my interests, I had always been a girly-girl. Why couldn't I wear makeup and cut open people's heads? Was neurosurgery really such a gendered concept? When you graduated, did they pass out stethoscopes and a beard trimmer?

Once again, I called my parents to hear what they would think. My mom had been doing progressively better, not quite but almost back to her old self. She wasn't anywhere near as passive as she had been the first year or so after her aneurysm. She said, in a solid voice, "Just do it, Sheri. And anyway," she added, ever ready with a relevant example, "think of those track athletes, the women who run very fast but also have their hair done, wear makeup, big necklaces, and have long nails. And they break world records. They're doing it their way, and it's not wrong. You do it your way, and it won't be wrong either. If you can still jump through all the hoops that you need to jump through, then who cares what you look like when you do it."

Ah, leave it to my mom. She would blindly support me no matter what. And I knew Alex would too.

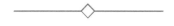

What it comes down to is this: you can talk to the people most important to you, the biggest experts in the field, and even they won't know what it's like to be you, how big and critical your dreams are, and what you can handle. I wasn't worried about Alex—we'd been through so much already that I knew unequivocally that we had each other's backs and could com-

municate clearly about our thoughts—but I saw that even his subtle bias-
es, from a different person, could have been enough to shake my resolve
if I had been either a little more uncertain or didn't have quite the same
support. Having faith in yourself means even—and especially—when you
aren't 100 percent certain of the path ahead. Go for the moon even without the guarantee your boots will touch the surface. You won't get far if
you wait for guarantees.

4

———

Find Your Way to Yes

Doing everything "right" and believing in yourself doesn't automatically guarantee you'll achieve your goals. Your dream can be thwarted by luck or chance or blocked by gatekeepers (or the occasional ogre). This doesn't mean there's no way through that gate.

You've mapped out your path to your goal, but that is your guide. To extend this metaphor, any good cartographer knows that roads may be added over the years, mountains can be tunneled through, or underground tunnels can be dug. Technology changes and adapts, and now there are even newer ways to get from Point A to Point B or C or Z.

The noes you might get are different from the naysaying; these are the people (or events) that directly block a passage through. Sometimes, you'll have to deal with them head-on; other times, you'll have to find a different way around. Gatekeepers are particularly insidious because they do hold the power to stop your path. Other times, events—catastrophic or traumatic or extremely difficult—will block your path and stall you for a while. It took eleven Apollo missions to actually make it to the moon, with a lot of astronauts who died following their dreams along the way. Imagine being a woman medical student in Afghanistan when the Taliban took over (either time). These are extreme examples, but yes, some roadblocks require more than just a reenergized stick-to-itiveness and grit.

Fortunately, for most of us, our roadblocks don't involve combustible rockets or governmental collapse. Still, it can be difficult to find a workaround for particularly nasty or vindictive ogres, but if your dream is important to you, it's important that you do find that workaround and not let a difficult person be the reason you don't make it to your own moon landing.

———————◇———————

I've witnessed plenty of inner-hospital gossip and backstabbing to the point I felt like I was back in middle school or in some playground for regressed adults. Throughout medical school, different factions fighting each other would separately try to pull me to their side. It was the most extreme in the surgery and surgical subspecialties, but I did experience some of it in Internal Medicine rotations as well.

One of the many instances occurred during my surgical rotation. I had the opportunity to perform a laparoscopic gallbladder resection and knew that I would likely face Monday morning "pimping," also called a Grand Rounds session, which is a cross between a football team watching Monday films of the weekend's game and hazing by the general surgery attending. I went to the residents' break room to review a chapter in my copy of *Netter*, an illustrative textbook owned by every single medical student across the country and the world, on the anatomy of the gallbladder and bile duct. All of a sudden, the door to the break room swung open, and Mirna walked in. *Stormed in* would be more appropriate.

Mirna was one of the senior residents, a tall and leggy Eastern European woman. I had seen her half an hour earlier when I was selected to scrub in for the surgery. The older residents were considered close to attendings, and I was awed by her and her level of seniority. She sat down at one of the computers, her back to me, and began to type furiously, pulling up patient charts. She sighed and swore, then banged her fist on the table. "Goddammit!"

She was completely unaware of my presence. I sat in the corner, sheepish, trying to bury my entire body behind my textbook. Mirna swore again, even louder this time, then turned her head enough to put me in her line of vision.

"Oh, sorry. You weren't supposed to hear that." She turned a light shade of red.

I wasn't sure what I should do. I was out of my comfort zone because this was a relatively intimate moment and yet there was this distance between her and me, a lowly medical student. I wasn't sure if I should ask her to share her thoughts. "What's wrong?"

She named the attending, saying his name with utmost disgust and adding an expletive. "He's making me round on patients again, and I want to operate." She had wanted in on the operation I would be assisting. Instead, the attending surgeon was making her do menial tasks and she was annoyed. She was beyond annoyed. "It's because I'm a girl. All the boys get to operate in their good ol' boys' club."

I nodded along, my eyes wide, feeling bad for her and making sure my expression communicated as much, holding back out of fear of saying the wrong thing. Mirna, however, was not one to hold back.

"Goddammit, I'm close to graduating. I really need to learn this case, and this asshole won't let me operate with him because I don't have a penis."

I tried to look exasperated with her, to match her mood, but without committing too much. I was swiftly learning that you had to play with the boys if you wanted to do these operations because if you didn't, you would get boxed out and the mostly male attendings would give the cases to somebody else. So, I had to roll with it and act like a guy—not lose my femininity, but I had to match them, play ball with them, in order to get the cases. It was exhausting, but I wasn't looking for a fight or crusade—all I wanted was to finish my rotation and not get roped into the politics of a place where I'd only be for a few more weeks.

I tried to keep my head down and roll with it, all while being memorable enough to be recognized and rewarded with surgical cases. All the medical students were walking a tightrope, but the women medical students were walking on a tightrope that was set on fire. I did my best to get the skills I needed while appearing as the team player with whichever disgruntled resident came to vent to me next. To say it was exhausting is an understatement. I told Mirna I was sorry, and I offered that it didn't seem fair.

"You'll see how it is—you have to watch your back around them," she said.

Mercifully for me, she went back to her work, and I was off the hook, at least temporarily. However, she had marked me as a sympathetic ear, and that would not be the last time Mirna would feel free to vent to me about her various injustices.

I did take note, though, of the names she dropped, the attendings who had boxed her out of surgeries. I'm sure I modified my behavior accordingly around these attendings. I wasn't into playing games, but I was going to keep doing whatever it took to get into those operating rooms and learn everything I could. I felt for Mirna, though—a woman who certainly didn't want to take no for an answer, but who, nevertheless, hit the brick wall of systemic unfairness.

I was not in a position to stand up for anything in this case, but there would be plenty of times I would be able to use my voice. It's also up to the doctors who do have power to speak up for others and give them a chance.

Many years later, I would witness a group of attendings stand up to an unethical doctor and remove him from the hospital. It was a shocking scene, but it was also gratifying and impressive, seeing the power to do right by the patients and other staff. For now, all I knew was that I had to bide my time until I did hold the power.

Some situations, of course, demand speaking out. I wished more of the attendings at Mirna's hospital had supported her. Her choosing to fight with them only made the gatekeepers holding her back lock her out further. She couldn't find her way around to a yes and was struggling.

That's the trick. We all want to be in a better world and to make a better world, but not everyone is in a position to fight every single battle. (It's even too much for a would-be tiger to fight battles on every front.) That makes it even more important to work in a spirit of cooperation, utilizing power as a collective, or just being there to help other people through the tough spots.

In the meantime, I was doing my best to thread the proverbial needle.

One way to find your way to yes? Have not just allies, but the people who will "get" you and your interests. Mirna needed an ally who wasn't just an intern she could vent to. She also needed someone who understood her no-nonsense sensibility. It's a hard case, and I'm certainly not going to say that the system was just or could easily have been bent to work in her favor. She needed help from someone who had actual power to help her, and that wasn't me back when I was a medical student.

It was at this time that I found not just allies but genuine supporters, and even the beginning of a circle of people who would change my life. Despite everyone who had dismissed my dreams in becoming a neurosurgeon, once I actually met and started working with neurosurgeons in my subspecialty rotation, the doctors there—all male—were nothing but supportive and encouraging. It was like being in a totally different world, despite being in the same hospital.

I got to know them all and followed them on their patient rounds and into the OR, where they walked me through the procedures. My gender, my skin color, these things never came up.

Dr. Peter, one of the neurosurgeons training me, sat me down on my fifth day and said, "If you want to do this job, this is the best job in the world. The reason is because you walk into the hospital, and everyone knows who you are, everyone respects you; you're not a doctor lost in the shuffle where nobody cares if you show up to work. What you do is so meaningful. Don't listen to all the pessimists and naysayers. You do your own thing, and you make your own decisions." Then he laughed. "You're really going to thank me some day. You're going to come back to me ten years from now and say, 'That jerk, he told me to become a neurosurgeon and this life sucks! And it's all because of him, and he sent me down the wrong path!'"

He was a goofy, hilarious, and smart guy—definitely not an ogre. If he drank his own pee, it certainly hadn't hurt him.

In fact, none of the four neurosurgeons were disgruntled or discouraging. The only naysayers had been people who weren't neurosurgeons. All the neurosurgeons loved their jobs and understood the enormity of what they were doing. By far, working with these doctors was the most fulfilling and enjoyable part of my entire medical school experience thus far.

Dr. Henry was one of the other neurosurgeons who provided so much support and guidance. While I was rotating at the hospital, an elderly woman was admitted from a nursing home. Her daughter brought her in, saying her mother hadn't been herself, and she was concerned because her mother hadn't been responding properly. Dr. Henry pulled up her CAT scan.

"Come over here and look at this, Sheri." He pointed his finger to the screen. "There are fluid collections on top of the brain—subdural hematomas. She may have fallen, or, because of the Coumadin she is taking, she may have bled into the brain." Either a fall or her blood thinners could be the culprit. "She probably needs to have these evacuated," Dr. Henry said to me.

As he sat down with the family members, I listened to the way he explained what this woman needed—artfully and diligently and with great patience—and her family understood. We booked the patient for surgery the next day.

The next morning, I woke up with a knot in my stomach. There was a good chance, and I was hopeful, that Dr. Henry would ask me to assist in the surgery. I had never held a surgical drill, the tool used to access the cranium. I was terrified.

I scrubbed my hands at the sink and then walked with Dr. Henry through the operating room doors. The patient was prepped and draped. Dr. Henry cut into the skin, explaining his process to me, showing me exactly what to look for. The bone was exposed, white and gleaming. Then, he turned to me. "Okay, you are going to do this." He handed me the drill. He showed me exactly where to make the first hole.

The drill was a pneumatic drill, operated by a foot pedal. I hit the pedal with my foot, and it whirred to life in my hand. Dr. Henry held my hand and pushed the drill into the bone. "Keep steady, keep steady." My hand wobbled as he supported it. Then he guided my hand to press deeper into the bone. "Hear that? That singing?" The drill was letting out a high whine. "That's when you're going through the cortical bone." All of a sudden, the drill abruptly stopped, and we were looking at the dura. That was the first burr hole that I ever drilled. "Thank you, Sheri, very nicely done."

I stepped back and watched as he finished the rest of the procedure. While we scrubbed out, I couldn't stop smiling.

"So?" Dr. Henry asked.

"That's it—I'm done. This is the only specialty that I can possibly choose."

Dr. Henry smiled too, nodding his head. He understood.

That surgery was the defining moment. I knew. I had found my circle.

There was one more thing I had to ask, and it came after the death of one of the patients I'd worked on with Dr. Peter. "How do you learn to deal with so much death?" It was the one thing that worried me about pursuing the neurosurgical life. How much of the death could I handle, of my everyday being the worst days of my patients' lives?

He nodded. "We do deal with a lot. They come to us because they're in really bad shape. You will be affected by patient deaths, some more than others. But you have to put up that wall, that emotional separation. You go in anyway. You do the job because there's even a slight chance of saving them or giving the patient more time. You can save them, and then they can go out and get hit by lightning. We can't control everything. We do our job, give them a chance. If not, we give them comfort and we give them dignity."

I nodded. It's what I already knew, but I was glad to hear it from a neurosurgeon I respected and admired.

"Do you have a good support structure?" Dr. Peter asked.

"Yes. My family is wonderful, and my partner has my back no matter what."

"Good, good. There will be tough times. You hold onto your life, your family. Your life can be neurosurgery, but your patients' lives, they aren't your life. If you can keep that up eight times out of ten, you'll do alright."

I took his words as gospel. Having other people with the same focus who understood who I was and would be going through on my path served as a polestar as things grew tougher, which they absolutely did during my residency.

Getting to my yes involved my support network and the people who got me, who were a like-minded community. The neurosurgeons wrote me glowing letters of recommendation when I applied for a competitive summer internship and then again when it came time to interview to "match" for residencies. However, there would still be barriers I'd have to find my way around.

How I would be matched with a hospital for my residency was far less poetic. The process by which residents are selected by a medical program, and vice versa, is through an outdated type of computer dating. We might as well have been swiping left or right.

The candidates first submit their information electronically to what was then called the San Francisco Match program. I uploaded medical school grades, boards scores, a personal photo, letters of recommendation, and "all other" activities, which entailed published articles, volunteering, and research involvement. Then, the programs would contact applicants for an interview, during which the candidate is questioned by the faculty in a one-on-one, two-on-one, or in rare cases, a three-on-one setting. The questions are meant to test the candidates' medical knowledge, and they range from simple, personal questions to complex medical queries in the style of an oral examination.

Then, either before or after the interview, the candidates are invited to a dinner with the residents and faculty. The dinner is a key component of the process; it's a chance to see how the faculty interact with their residents, revealing if they're too harsh with the residents or too soft, if they let the residents speak up, or if the residents are too intimidated. Also, since the dinners provide cocktails, the residents frequently "loosen up" after one or a few, and then their stories simply flow out like a tapped vein. The faculty and residents meanwhile get to talk with candidates in a less formal setting. Afterward, the candidates and the programs rank each other. This is based on a numeric scale; therefore, your first choice for residency is ranked #1, your second choice is #2, and so on. A candidate can only rank a program if they've had an interview with that program. All programs must be ranked and submitted by a deadline, and then the computer plugs and chugs the list of candidates and schools, and voilà! You've matched. Scratch the Tinder reference—the process is more like a sorority rush, but without all the singing. Each candidate matches with only one hospital, and it's all done during a matching ceremony which takes place at exactly the same time at every medical school across the United States.

Of course, not everyone gets matched. In that case, there is another process called "the scramble" in which a candidate has to find any open spots not already filled. At that point, it's a game of musical chairs.

Usually there are never any open spots in neurosurgery to scramble into. Neurosurgery's match rate is roughly 50 percent; half the candidates who apply will not match. So, finding your way to a yes is also about numbers. In that case, one of the options for candidates is to elect to spend the next year or two strengthening their application and then reapply to programs. At that point, some will match while others pursue other surgical subspecialties. (This is why mapmaking is such an important step to the self-actualization process.)

As I had learned and seen firsthand during my rotations in the last two years of medical school, residents are overworked and frequently stressed out, which can, and often does, lead to burnout. Some unfortunate souls sign up for the life of a brain surgeon and discover they can't handle the rigors, the pressures, or the death and so they drop out or pursue another field or choose a more "normal" existence without power tools in their everyday lives. Their moonshot dream turns out to be not exactly what they expected—and that's okay too. They gave it a shot. In those cases, their spots then open up to very relieved candidates for the residency who did not get an initial match.

I received eighteen offers for interviews, and I took sixteen of those. I would be traveling around the country to different health systems with each of them. What the medical rushing process set out to do came true; I did learn a lot about these hospitals and how they interacted with residents during the interviews.

I also learned a lot about how many hospitals felt about female neurosurgeons. Scratch that—the idea of a female neurosurgeon.

There are a few different types of special interview processes, and I was excited to have another sub-internship at a very high-powered university in the Midwest. One bonus was that I was invited to give a medical talk on aneurysms as a means of proving my qualifications, presenting a case with a patient in front of the whole group, including the senior staff neurosurgeon.

At the end of the sub-internship, when I went for my interview, I was greeted by the senior staff neurosurgeon. He was an older white man, balding, but his face was youthful. I had worked with him a number of times during my internship, and he'd seen me in action during my case presentation.

We sat down, and he perused my application, paging through the stack of papers. We started with small talk, as if having a dinner conversation at home, and I thought it was nice that we were chatting. I thought, *He's really using this one-on-one time, making an effort to know me better. This is good.*

But the chitchat and useless banter went on. Ten minutes, then fifteen, then twenty. We were like this for half an hour. I waited for the question about my goals in neurosurgery. I waited for him to ask if I would work hard and make the program proud. Then, he closed the paper stack and stared at me with his penetrating green eyes.

"You know," he said, "I see many things about you. You are affable, intelligent, hard-working, and bright."

I waited for the *but.* I held my breath, hanging on his next words.

"But neurosurgery is really only for white males."

He stood up abruptly to open his office door as I sat in the chair with my mouth agape. He gave a polite smile and nod to cover up the awkwardness, and I stood up and left.

It had never dawned on me that I would be discriminated against so obviously, so unapologetically, for both my ethnicity and gender. Perhaps it was how I was raised, perhaps it was having lived in so many different parts of the world, perhaps I didn't think in my profession someone who was highly qualified would be disqualified because of who she was. I had naively thought it couldn't happen in the neurosurgical field. I had even looked at Mirna's situation as something abstract, something that happened to somebody else, something that could happen to women if they didn't play the game. Now, it was real. Now, I understood it. Now, I deeply felt Mirna's frustration. It really could happen to any woman. I had never faced discrimination to this degree before. There had been a few elementary school playground incidents that I assumed were a common part of growing up with brown skin, but even these weren't horrible. Other children noticed the difference and asked why, and in high school, my sister and I were the only two Indian girls at our Catholic college preparatory academy, yet we were never made to feel less than anybody else. I had never been excluded because of my race or gender.

This man had accused me of two things that were true: I was a woman, and I was a first-generation US-born Indian American. These were facts—ones that I could not change.

There is a French expression, *l'esprit de l'escalier*, which translates to "spirit of the stairs," and it refers to thinking of the perfect witty retort to something only after it's too late to say it. I left his office without responding with a reply because I didn't have the words. I was twenty-seven years old, I had been through college, graduate school, medical school, and had devoted over a decade to my education, all toward becoming a neurosurgeon. In one tiny sentence, all my hard work had been reduced to nothing. My last month at that very hospital had just been reduced to nothing. All he saw were the two things he wanted to see about me, two things that shouldn't have mattered but that served to disqualify me for this residency, even after he'd seen the quality of the work I had done during my time at his hospital. That was perhaps the biggest betrayal.

I left feeling embarrassed and ashamed. A true tiger would have had a much different reaction. She would have given a man like that the business end of her claws.

I rushed back to the hotel to call Alex.

"How'd it go?" He answered the phone cheerfully. "It should have been a piece of cake—you spent an entire month there. They know you well."

In that instant, it dawned on me. Alex had never been disqualified because of his gender. The world really is a different place for men than it is for women. If Alex had been in my shoes, that senior neurosurgeon would have asked him all about his goals, would have remarked on the presentation he'd given to the department, maybe even would have asked Alex on for the residency. Alex never would have known that neurosurgeon was a misogynist.

"Well . . . it wasn't exactly what I expected," I said.

"What do you mean? What did they ask you to do? Perform brain surgery?" He laughed at his own joke.

"The attending surgeon told me not to bother ranking the program. That I would never get in because I was not white and male."

There was a slight pause, as if what I said needed to register with Alex. "He said that? Really?"

"Yep."

"You can't say stuff like that."

"True, but he did." My shock and embarrassment were tinted now with anger.

Alex sighed. "Better to know now rather than be stuck there for seven years."

"You're right." I was tired, let down, frustrated. I had gained so much knowledge and experience, and I had always believed that knowledge was power. I had seen it in action. But in this instance, that knowledge wasn't enough, and I was powerless. Why had they even invited me to interview in the first place if they knew they weren't going to take me? *Oh*, I realized, *so they could say they interviewed women candidates and let them give presentations. I was just a quota so they could avoid getting into trouble.* "I guess that month was a complete waste of time."

"Hey, listen," Alex said. "You need to take a chance. You know you can do it. You should bet on yourself."

Bet on myself. I felt as if a giant bell had been rung inside of me—a deep, resonating sound. I would bet on myself. Despite that attending surgeon's stature, despite his exceptional skills, despite the highest level of respect he received from his peers, I saw him as small. What a small man to see the world in that way. What a small man to make such a sweeping, let alone discriminatory, statement. What a small man to not give someone else a chance. What a small man for seeing all my qualifications on paper and rule me out because I dared to sit in his office with brown skin and a woman's body.

It would take years of experience and reflection for me to understand that some of my paralysis came from how much power I lacked in that situation. He was a gatekeeper. Was I supposed to chew him out and run the risk of him sharing how "difficult" I was with the other neurosurgical programs? I played scenes in my mind involving my name at the top of a blacklist circulated among the (very small) neurosurgical world.

I decided not to rank the program at all. However, that presentation I gave absolutely went on my curriculum vitae. I would use it to bet on myself somewhere else. There were plenty of other places where I could thrive.

Unfortunately, those places were more difficult to find than I thought.

There were other interviews, mostly in the South, where I was told that women shouldn't bother applying because they'd never accept a female resident, despite what my application may boast or who had written my letters of recommendation. They didn't mention the color of my skin, but at that point, what did it matter? As I crisscrossed half of the country, meeting other candidates during the process, I'd come across fifteen or so women; we'd nod to each other in solidarity. Chatting over glasses of wine at the dinners, I heard of many more stories from the few other women-neurosurgical hopefuls that my experiences were not unique.

We had a special camaraderie, the other women applying for neurosurgical residencies. Though we rarely saw each other, when we did, we always made sure to approach each other, say hello and shake hands, and if we had time, chat about our experiences on the interview trail. I learned how many other universities had rejected them based on their gender. I was glad for not wasting my time by applying to many of these other schools, though I'd had my share of them as well. It was sobering news.

When I got to Rhode Island for my interview at Brown University, my first choice because of its outstanding residency program for neurosurgery, I was horrified to learn I was one out of eighty candidates interviewing over a period of two days for the one spot. One out of eighty? There were seventy-nine other well qualified candidates vying for this neurosurgical residency? Still, this was my dream program, and I was betting on myself. I considered my odds: my application was competitive, and I had received seventeen other interview offers, which was a good number—an auspicious sign, I hoped.

Brown had indeed had a woman neurosurgical resident, but she had graduated thirteen years earlier. There hadn't been a woman since. It was a shocking statistic, but it also signaled to me that it was past time they had another woman, and that should be me.

Bet on myself. Bet on myself. I was determined to find my way to a yes.

The chairman who conducted my interview was a lovely and cordial elderly gentleman, who most importantly sounded passionate about neurosurgical residency training.

"You have an impressive application," he told me. I held my breath. This hospital was so wonderful. I didn't want the other shoe to drop. "I very much enjoyed reading about your graduate degree research. It seems like there would be a lot you could bring to the hospital."

Then, the woman administrator who had led the tour asked me my marital status. I held my breath.

"I will be getting married this summer."

"And have you considered what the residency would do to your upcoming marriage?" the chairman added. "What will your husband do while you're working?" The chairman didn't sound condescending. It didn't feel like some kind of trap or disqualifier.

"Alex can stand on his own two feet—he always has. After obtaining a PhD in biochemistry from Northwestern University, I'm not too worried about his potential research prospects." Of course, we would find a way to make it all work.

The chairman smiled at my answer. He and the other two interviewing me nodded to each other. He then talked more about the program, about the strong community of neurosurgeons at Brown, and he asked me what it was I liked best about neurosurgery. We had a real conversation. Everything he said was delivered with a fatherly but non-condescending tone. My gender never came up.

I left the interview ecstatic. It had gone well, I had brought my best, and I was already feeling like I fit the program and the hospital so well. I could imagine spending the next seven years there. All my hopes had been confirmed. My concerns were the other seventy-nine medical students who were qualified to be there.

On Match Day, when it came time to open all our white envelopes, I found out that I had matched with Brown, my dream school.

It is difficult even now to put into words the kind of absolute triumph I felt, especially as Alex bear-hugged me, and my parents, teary-eyed, swarmed me. I would imagine it's what the climbers of Everest feel when they summit or when astronauts step onto the launch pad at Cape Canaveral. The feeling of taking on the hardest task imaginable and accomplishing it. I would be the first woman neurosurgical resident at Brown in an entire generation. It felt monumental.

My mapped route to becoming a neurosurgeon had to go through a residency program; I wanted Brown, that was my ideal route, but by no means was it the only route. Had I not matched with Brown but another residency, I would also have found my way to yes. Had I not matched at all, I would have tried again the next year. Once I had my neurosurgical subspecialty rotation and drilled a burr hole, I knew it was the path for me. It was no longer theoretical. So yes, by whatever means, I would have found my way to a residency. I learned that a no was merely a temporary situation I could get around.

My mom regularly quoted Martin Luther King, Jr., and other civil rights leaders, telling me to always keep my eye on the prize, to not get distracted or derailed by roadblocks. Those would be bound to happen, but if it was something urgent that I staked my life on, that was going to be important to me for my whole life. Then one way or another, as long as I kept my focus on that goal, I could reach it.

She knew well about detours and taking other doors. Her story was my earliest example of finding a way to yes, even though I didn't realize it at the time.

My mother had always been in academia, but when I was young, my father moved around for work—Illinois; Seoul, South Korea (when I was a baby); Houston and Beaumont in Texas; and then my father was recruited as a project engineer for the oil company Aramco in Dhahran, Saudi Arabia. The company had its own Western expatriate housing compounds and provided us housing as part of my father's contract. The compound was its own city, fifty-eight kilometers long (larger than some countries). Inside the compound walls, life was like any other American suburban city, with neighborhood streets and shopping centers called commissaries, looking more like a city in Illinois or Texas than Saudi Arabia.

On the weekends, my family would head to the beach on the Arabian Gulf, dodging jellyfish in the warm water. We relished swimming in the deep jewel-toned sea, playing in the sand dunes, returning home to hot showers and lazy evenings. Sometimes I could get Jiji to pretend with me that we were animals, although she didn't care for animals as much as I did. I always wanted to be a tiger. Even at the beach, when Jiji scoffed that tigers didn't hang out at the beach, I insisted that they could swim, so it didn't matter where we played. I roared on the dunes, I roared in the hallways of our house on the compound, I roared in the bathtub, queen of all my domain, relatively untouched by the world around me.

It didn't take me long to notice the difference between life on the compound, which was comprised entirely of Americans or Europeans, and life off the compound. On the compound, my mother would drive us around to the stores and wear Western clothing, which was the only kind of clothing I had ever seen her wear. Off the compound, though, I began to realize there was a distinction between men and women in terms of gender and the expectations that came with those gender distinctions. Off the compound, my mother had to relinquish the wheel, and it was my father who sat in the driver's seat. My sister and I were young, not even teenagers yet, so we could wear whatever we wanted, whether on or off the compound. We typically wore skirts and t-shirts, and nobody paid any mind to us. But to leave the compound, my mother had to wrap her hair in a scarf in the style of a hijab, tie it at the nape of her neck, and don the long *abaya*, a kaftan-like cloak to cover her arms and legs. Large sunglasses covered her eyes. My mother couldn't go off-compound alone, without my father or a group of women.

My mom was hired by Aramco as a "casual employee," which was the official title. This title was given to women because Saudi law prohibited the hiring of female employees. As a casual employee, she worked on and off in an administrative capacity. She was a personnel administrator at one point, then she worked in an office as an administrative assistant. Though she had her master's degree, and technically was working, my mother took a hit professionally by being away from her ongoing research—her real work—for so long. Her career had taken a back seat to my father's because we had moved to such a restrictive environment. But it had been too good an opportunity for my family to pass up.

"Don't you miss your old job?" I asked her one day when she was talking about her ideas on a research project she wanted to take on in the future, which would examine the Indian diaspora and how they impact the political system throughout the United States.

"I do, and I will go back. That's still who I am, that won't ever change." She brushed the back of her hand against my cheek. "Don't ever forget, Sheri, if you want to be something in your life, if you want to do something, you are the only one who can stop you. A truly determined person will always find a way. It might not be immediately. That doesn't mean we don't prepare in the meantime."

Early on in our stay in Dhahran, I was diagnosed with asthma at the compound clinic. "I don't know what the trigger is," the Saudi doctor said. "It could be allergies." We didn't have a family history of asthma or allergies. I had to return to the clinic many times for nebulizer treatments—sometimes with the same doctor, sometimes with others. All of them were men. Finally, one day, as one of the doctors was loading the serum into the nebulizer, I asked him, "Do you have any lady doctors?"

His head shot up, and he almost laughed. "Oh, no, no, no, no. Not here. We don't need women to be doctors in Arab countries." He blew off the idea as not just custom but as something ridiculous.

Jiji and I learned to accept that there were places in the world that imposed different codes of living just because you were a woman and not a man. That's how life was where we grew up, but I also understood that it didn't have to be that way for me. That on the compound, women were mostly free to do what they wanted. That's how I thought life should be. It bothered me though that there couldn't be a woman doctor on the compound. If it was on the compound, what did it matter who treated patients? I was especially incredulous when that system affected me personally. My mom had bought Jiji and me a very expensive anatomy book. After all the talk about my lungs and visits to the doctor, I was enthralled with learning more about the body, and I wanted to see all my parts diagrammed in detail. I imagined the pages would have the layers of transparencies, where I could flip up the top page, which had the skin, revealing the next layer of nerves, flipping again to reveal the muscles and the organs, and finally, the skeleton. My mom ordered it from a special bookstore and had it shipped to us at the compound. When it arrived, all the images containing skin had been blackened out, painstakingly, with black marker. Every beautiful illustration and image wiped out with heavy ink. Saudi Arabia censored even the body on the page in a medical text-book. *What did their doctors do?* I wondered. I felt cheated and beyond disappointed. My mom tried to be pragmatic about it, but the book and the shipping had been expensive and even she was miffed.

As Jiji and I grew older, we left Saudi Arabia so that we wouldn't have had to be sent away to boarding school due to lack of high school options. We ended up at my grandmother's house in India where I continued my asthma treatment in a horrific hospital that did not have the funds or the pristine spotlessness of the Saudi hospital. The halls and rooms were dimly lit, with few windows. Everything was dirty, especially the floors, which were covered in various types of filth, most of which I didn't want to know anything about. The staff seemed chaotic, and there was no orderliness to how the patients were managed. The equipment looked old-fashioned compared with what I saw in Saudi Arabia.

The one constant from Saudi Arabia, though? All the doctors were men. There were women working at the hospital, at least, but they were all nurses (and there were no nurses who were men) and the doctors made it as much their practice to talk down to the nurses, dictating to them and patronizing them, as the actual practice of treating patients. These doctors made me nervous; the hospital made me queasy. I was grateful for the constant presence of Jiji during my half-hour nebulizer treatments. She would have her nose in a book on Egyptology or her new love, as-tronomy, but would tap my knee every so often to make sure I was okay. As long as she was there, I was okay—that became my mantra. I wasn't okay with much else, especially when one of the doctors told my mom my asthma was becoming a chronic problem. (I had to ask Jiji what *chronic* meant. She said that it meant I'd have to deal with asthma my whole life, probably.) Even worse, I was prescribed Theophylline, a type of asthma medication in common use that made me (and many other people) sick to my stomach. Eventually, it was no longer used due to side effects. Thus, my time in India was completely miserable, physically and emotionally.

After a few months, my mom and dad quickly realized that India was no longer the place for them, that it was no longer their home, and finally they announced to us that we would be moving back to Illinois. No, my asthma didn't miraculously clear up when I got back, but it was manageable and my new doctor's office at the nearby hospital was much more like Dhahran: clean and sterile, with even a few doctors who were women walking around. It was a major culture shock to go back to the United States after so many years abroad. I started school in the middle of the school year, on my tenth birthday, so I was both excited and nervous. My teacher introduced me, saying, "Class, our new student, Sheri, has just moved here from Saudi Arabia."

A kid in the front looked at me quizzically. "Where's Saudi Arabia?"

How could he not know? There were Americans in Saudi Arabia. Was I so different? Apparently, I was.

"You talk funny," another kid said at recess. I didn't know how I talked. I didn't talk like the kids in India. I didn't speak like a Saudi kid. I sounded a lot like the kids on the compound, and I sounded just like my sister. I'd never thought I spoke funny before. I began at this age to think of myself more as a child of the world, a global citizen, than someone who was from any one place. I was now living in my fourth country, the one that was supposedly home, but it didn't yet feel that way. I thought, *The world is an awfully big place. Is there just one home for a person?* It took a while but eventually I wasn't the friendly girl who was from a weird place and talked funny, but just the friend Sheri from school. Through all of these changes, my one constant was Jiji. As long as I had my sister, I was okay. She was the saving grace of my childhood. Having Jiji around ensured that I was never by myself at a lunch table, that I wasn't the only one going through the culture shock.

"You're both brave girls," my mother told us, matter-of-factly. She reminded us again that our lives were still very fortunate. No whining, in other words. My mother wasn't being unsympathetic, either. Her approach was to put things in perspective. And we were now back in a country where I could read whatever anatomy book I wanted, with all the pictures.

And back in Illinois? My mom went back for another degree and embarked on her teaching career that started her on the path to being the woman of the year, Human Dynamo. The roadblock was only temporary. She found her way to yes, just as she would in recovering from her aneurysm. She was forced into early retirement, but she found her way back to most of the other things she loved. We were privileged enough to be able to move around, but that's also what our family had to be willing to do in order to have the life we all wanted. It's also how I had faith when applying to neurosurgical residencies that I would make it work, one way or another.

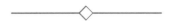

I think of those women in Saudi Arabia, even in certain places in India, who can't be doctors, or have the jobs they want, or drive a car. Their roads to yes are much harder than what most of us go through. People living in a war-torn country or extreme poverty with no way to get out of it, for many of them, it can be condescending to say, "Follow your dream!" when there are structural factors in place that make it nearly impossible. That doesn't mean impossible in every case. (One has to only look back at historic trailblazers and movements that have led to political and social revolutions.) If you're reading this book, though, you probably have considerably more agency over your own life. Hold on to that.

Even amid a detour, don't think of it as wasted time. Do with it what you can because our time, after all, is precious, and the detour may just lead you to another way of getting to your yes. What you have to watch out for is letting yourself get sidetracked on too many detours, which can carry you far away from your goal. If your goal changes, that's one thing; plot your new coordinates from that point on. If you do find yourself getting too far away from where you do want to be, that's the time to go back to the map and recenter yourself.

5

Hold On to What Drives You:
The "P" Words

If I hadn't loved neurosurgery, the beauty of it, there was no way I could have gotten through the rigors and the early horrors and frustrating cases I experienced during residency. My medical school colleague, Roger, comes to mind every so often—the one who thought it would be "cool" to be an orthopedic surgeon but didn't like surgery. How could he possibly face going into work in a very difficult career track, investing so much time and energy into something he didn't like? How might it affect his patients if he couldn't get over his squeamishness?

I don't know what happened to Roger, maybe it all "clicked" into place, and he found his love for it after all. Familiarity can do a lot to give you appreciation and even love. However, if you can't find your way to being *passionate*, that can be a bad sign for overall well-being.

It sounds trite, but think about what gets you up in the morning, what makes you excited for a new day. What are you waking up for? Use that road map to know what the end goal is and that getting up, not procrastinating on the steps, will get you to that end goal one day faster. There was purpose every time I forced myself to wake up and go into another long stretch of running around the hospital, treating trauma after trauma, on my feet for hours straight with no food or water, and then filling out endless paperwork, sometimes multiple times if I made a mistake (such as using blue ink instead of black). There were stretches I was so tired I envied my trauma patients because they got to lie down. (Exhaustion really skews perspective, sometimes.) However, being in the operating room drove me; it was what I loved, and it was where I belonged. I needed that passion to get me through the hardest times.

Doing anything hard will push you and challenge you, and if you discover the passion and love for it isn't there, you may wonder whether that dream is for you after all. However, if you do love it, you will need to hold on to that passion for the really hard days. Some days, that might be all that gets you through.

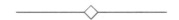

July first is the worst time to go to a teaching hospital because that's the date when all the fresh residents start. Fourth of July would mark my first overnight call in neurosurgical training. It also happened to be the busiest day of the year for neurotrauma in Rhode Island. Fourth of July served as a hazing ritual for the incoming neurosurgical resident. As the senior residents looked on, I was the newbie who was the proverbial "deer in the headlights." Figuratively, but as close to literally as you could get.

Much like hazing for fresh residents, Rhode Islanders also had their Independence Day rituals they ascribed to. Rhode Island is populated by citizens loyal to Roger Williams, the man who founded the state based on the concept of defense from religious persecution and other such infarctions. Essentially, there aren't a lot of laws in place designed to infringe upon one's civil liberties. Because of this tradition and his legacy, there was no such law requiring motorcyclists to wear helmets. Winters in Rhode Island can be hairy for motorists, but one of the things that make neurosurgeons cringe is when the warm weather moves in. More people go out in warm weather, riding their motorcycles, with their God-given right to feel the wind blow through their hair without being impeded by the civil prison that is a motorcycle helmet. Unfortunately, drinking and driving go hand in hand with the warmer months. So, whenever it was warm outside, and we were on-call, we knew it would be notoriously busy. Now magnify that by twenty and you'd have Rhode Island on the Fourth of July weekend.

That first Fourth of July, I had twenty-one consults. All the shock trauma rooms in the emergency room were filled with neurosurgical cranial and spinal emergencies. Pathologies ranged from head bleeds because of simple mechanical falls to spinal cord trauma with ensuing paralysis.

All hands were on deck; the nurses were at the top of their game that day, keeping watchful eyes on all new surgical residents as we performed invasive procedures such as external cranial drains and central lines.

The resident pager trilled at an alarming rate, every ten or fifteen minutes a new consult, a new request, an update. We ran short on beds in the neurosurgical ICU and so had to fill the medical and trauma units on the third and fifth floors with our patients, which generated even more pages. The nursing staff on those floors were less familiar with neurosurgical patients, and they wanted additional confirmation on their assessments and explanations for the unique orders.

Around 6:00 p.m., the dust finally settled in the emergency room, and a calm was palpable throughout the hospital. Busy residents finished consultation notes, last minute orders, and discussions with patients' families. I went through my list of forty patients and ensured that all tasks had been addressed: labs checked, orders reviewed, imaging noted. I was grateful for a moment to sit down. Despite my comfortable surgical clogs, I had been running back and forth to the ER so many times that the painful ache and fatigue had long set into my feet.

Then, the pager chimed. I answered the call.

"Hello, Dr. Dewan, Neurosurgery, returning a page."

"Oh, yes, hello. This is Dr. Stephens, one of the ER residents." She also would have been a new resident, just starting this week. There was a familiar methodical cadence to her voice, mixed with shell shock. Also, deductive reasoning: she was working on the holiday. "I have a new consult for you in Trauma 5. It's a young woman who was lighting off fireworks today at Federal Hill—" she paused. "Well, I guess . . . one was faulty. She picked it up to see if it was lit, and, well, it was."

I listened, wondering what the neurosurgical issue could be. Did she have a head injury? Brain bleeding? A fall resulting in spine trauma? The possibilities were lengthy.

"I think you should just come down and see her," Dr. Stephens said. "She is in Trauma 5."

"May I ask what the neurosurgical issue is? Head injury, spine? Has she had any imaging?" I wanted more details to prepare a course of action.

Dr. Stephens, the young resident, seemed even more deer in the headlights than I did. "Well—well, please just come down," she stammered. "I don't know all the neurosurgical terminology, but in brief, she blew out her eye, there is brain coming out of her nose, spinal fluid is leaking on her pillow, and her optic nerve looks severed." The timbre of her voice rose. "The eyeball is gone. It's just gone."

I hung up the phone and jumped onto the closest computer to pull up her CT scans. Though I was still a novice, it was evident. She sustained extensive cranial and skull trauma. The frontal bone and base of skull were shattered, and there was air inside the brain, indicating a bidirectional conduit—the hole was allowing a general coming in and going out of fluid, air, and potential infectious matter. I raced down to the ER, the route I'd already taken multiple times that day.

Trauma 5 was filled with medical staff in every color of scrubs. As soon as I entered the room, everyone stopped moving. All eyes were on me to watch my examination of the patient, waiting for my assessment of the damage. The patient was intubated with a breathing tube and heavily sedated. I grabbed a flashlight to examine her pupillary reflexes, test her corneal response, as well as her cough and gag. Her right eye was gone. Completely gone. No trace of it. As if it vanished into thin air on Federal Hill. Possibly incinerated in the blast. Her brain was herniating through the eye defect, the tissue and parenchyma (the functional tissue) bloodied and swollen. Spinal fluid dripped onto her cheek. The optic nerve had been severed at the root. Based on her reactions, her motor strength was impaired, with minimal movement.

The next few hours were a whirlwind of phone calls, arrangements with teams of consultants and constant updates to her family members. Apparently, it hadn't been an actual firework that had done the damage. They had started making and setting off Molotov Cocktails, which are illegal throughout the United States.

That night, once we lined up a plan of action, I was part of a team of neurosurgeons, ophthalmologists, and plastic surgeons set to perform an eighteen-hour procedure. While most people were enjoying time with their family and friends, chatting, watching fireworks, then going to sleep in their down comforters, we fought to save this patient's life. And the patient fought to save herself.

She made it through surgery, and I drove home, exhausted. At best, the patient would need extensive rehabilitation. She was a fighter, but prognostics were so tricky. *What gives life meaning?* I asked myself. *At what point is someone better off dead than alive if they're in a near-vegetative state?* It wasn't for me to decide, though. It had been my responsibility to try to help save her. I did everything in my power to do so. What could I do though against all the people who would put themselves into harmful situations, time and again, the kind of situations that leave a permanent pit in a surgeon's stomach?

As I pulled into the driveway of our townhouse, I thanked my lucky stars that my body and brain were intact, functioning and connected. Alex was waiting for me when I walked through the door and as I collapsed on the couch.

The patient spent two months in the hospital. A permanent feeding tube and breathing tube were placed. She was eventually transferred to a long-term care facility for extensive rehabilitation. I never saw her again, and I heard nothing about her recovery or survival beyond that. To this day, I wonder what happened to her.

I mention this case because it was part of a long streak of seeing catastrophic injury day in and day out, being exhausted, and wondering if what I was doing was the right thing. The other neurosurgeons reminded me that was the job. I knew this in my heart, but my mentors, especially the senior neurosurgeon, Dr. Cahill, encouraged me to be passionate about the fighting, about the brain, about the work of the job and giving the patient the best possible outcome that could be achieved with our skill.

The repeated theme of a neurosurgeon's life: it's upsetting to spend so much time and effort trying to save someone who may be beyond saving. You want to hope for patients. As a surgeon, you have to hope for patients; it's the way to ensure you are always doing the best you possibly can for them. You have to shut off everything else except for doing your job. Prognosticating ends when you scrub in. Do we hope for miracles? Do I believe in miracles? I have certainly seen the miraculous, but my experience has taught me not to count on the miraculous. That's emotional thinking, and it is too costly for neurosurgeons and probably many other surgeons as well. It certainly was the case with Dr. Stephens, whom I would work with for the next six years. She, too, found her way through the difficult first years by being passionate about the work, and by the time she graduated, she was a calm and in-control doctor at the top of her game.

"You know, Sheri," Dr. Cahill said one shift, "neurosurgery is the loneliest profession. In our work, we won't always get to have a team. We're alone, many times, dealing with making the toughest decisions, making split-second decisions for the life of somebody else, and there will be no one to turn to at four in the morning. It is a big burden that's often solely on our shoulders."

It was. I reminded myself that tigers were solitary creatures.

His words didn't solve the problem of the loneliness, except that if we knew other neurosurgeons, we knew we were part of a collective of people who saw the world the same way. Who, with a look, got exactly what we were going through. By even sitting down with me, I felt the connection amid our two lonely selves.

"You're a good neurosurgeon," he said. "Remember that. We save people, even if we can't solve all of human misery. No one can do that."

Though I was confident in my skills, I still wrestled every day with my own doubts about myself, my abilities to hang tough in this life. Another resident had recently left, gone to a different specialty. What Dr. Cahill said reinforced what I'd been using to keep myself going: neurosurgery was my purpose. Thinking back to my mother's recovery from her aneurysm and stroke, it was crystal clear to me that I was put on this earth to save other mothers, fathers, family members, loved ones.

Purpose is a powerful asset. It's the magus guiding you on your path, the talisman against the darkness, the power that lies at the center of everything you do. If you find your purpose, that makes everything easier. Once you know your purpose, the decision making is done. You commit and then you complete. It is the light that in any mistake illuminates the way forward, the lesson learned, so that the mistake doesn't repeat itself. Purpose fuels ambition to succeed, despite the greatest of odds. When something is your purpose, there's no fighting against it.

Not everyone will understand your drive and your purpose, and that's okay—you have to navigate that as well. Residency pushed me harder than even medical school had. I wasn't sleeping. I was overworked. I was seeing the worst sorts of traumas. However, if I confided about how miserable I was physically during my residency to either Alex or my parents, they would be worried for me, and I didn't want to put that kind of burden on them. Also, many times during residency I saw things that were beyond horrendous but couldn't share them with my biggest supporters. I tried once to explain a rough trauma that had come into the ER with Alex, and he was too grossed out to hear about it. There was a loneliness to that realization, that the person who had my back the most could not fully embrace my experience with me. Alex was even a biologist, so the body was not a foreign concept to him.

It was the same with my sister. Jiji was a constant supporter of my life, but even she regularly accused me of being weird. Sure, she could lean into both supporting me while also ribbing me, such as when she went to Cuzco and brought me back a two-hundred-page book on Peruvian trepanation, the Incan practice of rudimentary brain surgery. Yes, she was calling me out for being weird, but I absolutely loved my souvenir.

She and I talked regularly while I was in my residency, and one morning after I got off a twenty-four-hour call, up all night operating, she called and asked about my morning.

"There was a gunshot wound to the head, and this young kid, he was targeted by the South Providence gangs. I had to take these bullet fragments out of his head this morning. Every time I removed a piece, I had to hand it off to a police officer who was scrubbed in and waiting next to me with an evidence bag."

I waited a moment, and Jiji didn't respond. I heard a sip through a straw, sounding like the slurping of the bottom of a smoothie she'd had for lunch. "You know what I did today?" she said. "I went to the gym and got a coffee because that's what normal people do."

"Well, normal people who aren't brain surgeons," I said.

"Sheri, your life is not normal." She laughed, and she was right. For most people. I had chosen the weird and beautiful and complicated path of cutting up, picking at, fixing up people's brains.

I was tired, though. I wanted to be normal, to go to the gym and have a coffee and work maybe long but normal hours, like Jiji, and if I had to take work home with me, it wasn't life or death. I wanted to be able to go out with Alex any night we felt like it. I didn't want to have to plan my life around on-call shifts.

But being away from the operating room itself? No. That was the part I loved. What I was passionate about. I wouldn't give that up for anything in the world.

I worried, though, that something was wrong with me. Why did I love surgery so much?

What bothered me about my occupation, aside from the grueling residency part, had been witnessing organs removed from the body for harvesting or an autopsy. It was the dismantling of the body's form that went against my every impulse and instinct. When it came to the drills and the blood and the details of life preserving? I thrived off the energy of it, how close it put me to the absolute edge of what humans can do, even though it was still messy and ill-finessed because I didn't yet have all the techniques embedded in my fingers from years of experience. Maybe Jiji was right. Maybe I wasn't normal.

However, Dr. Cahill was always there to remind me that, while what we do isn't normal, we're the ones who have chosen to do this, we're needed, our work is important, and if we can hang on and understand that, we can tackle any problem. Though it was hard, I could deal with things that most people could not, even Alex and Jiji. Despite having gagged at the sight of my mother trickling spinal fluid into her coffee, now I could get past those horrors to do what needed to be done. Dr. Cahill and every other neurosurgeon were proof that it could be done, so why not me? Even the Incans could do it.

Every career path will have its oddities, the things only understood by the cadre of people who make up that world. That's okay if they're the ones who really get you. What's most important is that you have the faith in yourself and belief that you are in the right place and that you deserve to be there. Feel that purpose and let it ignite your passion. That's your fuel.

Jiji called us neurosurgeons weird. I think part of that stems from adapting for survival. We can't emotionalize, so instead, we focus on the brain. It is about the brain as much as possible. I'm aware of who these patients are, what families they have, what chances they each have when they come across the table, but surgery is mechanical. If it were a matter of keeping tally, a sort of wins or losses against death, we would likely lose ourselves in despair. The sad truth is that the odds are not good for many of our patients—that's why they come to us. But then I think of my mother. She'd survived the odds of even making it to the hospital. She'd survived the aneurysm, stroke, and vasospasm, and Dr. Johnson had kept her alive. She had suffered a loss of cognition, and though she would never be what she once had been and still struggled to remember dates or faces—my mother had always been so good at recognizing faces—she was able to regain much of her old self and come back from the proverbial dead.

It is estimated that tiger hunts are only successful about one in every ten or twenty attempts. I could do better than those odds. So maybe I would work for the off chance of a miracle.

That was, aside from loving the work, the purpose I found in the work. Every day that I dragged myself out of bed, not only did I love the work, but I knew there were patients relying on the work I did each and every day.

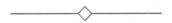

It doesn't matter what you do. It doesn't have to be about saving lives or changing the world. The importance of being passionate and finding your purpose isn't limited to neurosurgery. Passion helps focus the energy of your work, and it goes hand in hand with finding meaning (and purpose) with the work.

Another important point is that not everyone ends up having the dream version of the dream job. Does that mean not to map it? Not to shoot for the big goal? Absolutely not. Likewise, don't get derailed if expectations don't match reality. If your dream is to be the next Meryl Streep, really think about what that means. To have her career? To have her list of awards? Or to be as good an actor as Meryl Streep? Being a world-famous actor is an enticing goal, to be sure, but some of it boils down to luck and timing on top of the hard work. However, to be as good? That takes practice and dedication. Studying the craft of it. That's all 100 percent controllable. Maybe you become the Meryl Streep of community theater. Regional theater. Off-off Broadway. Most people with careers like Streep's devote themselves to the craft of acting, as opposed to seeking the fame and celebrity or accolades that can sometimes come with the career. That doesn't mean to stop trying for that great film role, but it also means not to be crushed by every role not gotten, every audition that didn't go your way. Don't derail yourself because what you want isn't happening exactly the way or at the pace of your dream. Instead, focus on what you can do in the present. Focus on the steps on your map.

There were plenty of people I knew from medical school who didn't match with a neurosurgical residency (or a residency of their choice). Sometimes they tried again the following year and matched; other times, they found their way to a different surgical specialty. And they thrived there.

Another important point: if you don't find a way to thrive in what you do for a living, find an outlet that gives you purpose and ignites your passion. Maybe you take an eight-to-five job purely for the financial aspect, but it's also a job you can leave behind at the end of the working day, allowing you to pursue your dream interests. You take a less-than-dream job because it gives you freedom to spend time on doing what you do love the rest of the time. Community theater, perhaps? Maybe it's traveling, volunteering, writing, playing music, an adult dodgeball league. Passion can look like a lot of things. Alex thought he'd found a great career path in biotech when we first moved to Rhode Island, but what he loved was biological research and sharing that with enthusiastic students. He found his way to that through teaching at a local college and doing a postdoctoral fellowship, and every day he could get up and go in because he was passionate about the work.

The key is that along with being passionate, be intentional. Keep the fire for what you love however you can. Map what you want, find your way around obstacles, and let your passion and purpose drive you.

6

———

Put a Pin in It

Passion and purpose can help drive you through some of the hardships you'll experience on the way to achieving your goal, but they aren't cure-alls. You can put your head down and your nose to the proverbial grindstone when necessary. Sometimes bad things happen, and you can't adequately address the trauma in the moment because you have to focus on the job at hand (this is familiar to all medical and rescue workers, and I'm sure many others).

It's one thing to push down some of the emotions in dealing with workplace traumas, but that doesn't mean to never deal with the emotions that stem from them. In many different areas, we will all see awful things and experience traumas along the way. There's so much of our collective lives filled with horrible things (as all of us post-2020 have seen). Be patient and kind with yourself, but deal with the emotions before they swallow you. Know when to put the trauma aside, but be sure to come back to really deal with the emotional aftereffects.

———◇———

Neurosurgical residents have a high burnout rate, stemming largely from dealing with so much day in and day out, made worse by not taking the time to eventually process the emotional aspects of the job. Unfortunately, neurosurgeons also can't let that interfere with the job of saving people's lives. The task is twofold: dealing with some of the most gruesome injuries and then dealing with times when, despite all our hard work, the patient doesn't survive. All surgeons have to try, even in the face of the impossible, to give the patient a fighting chance. Some injuries will be too critical and beyond even the skill of the best surgeon. Losing patients never becomes rote; we surgeons internalize all of that. The key that I learned is to put a pin in the horror and the death that I was confronted with daily; deal with the task first, but then process the emotions once the job is done.

It's not a perfect system, as it really is unfortunate that so many otherwise qualified people burn out, and part of that is the hazing of residents and just how few of them are around to do the work. Early on, I had to work with a 103-degree fever, but when I called the chief resident and told him that I could barely stand, after the briefest of pauses, he said, "Just push through it, Sheri. We have fifty-five patients to round on today. We have four operating rooms going. We just need you—there's no time to get sick."

Residents don't get sick days. I pulled myself out of bed to the sounds of Alex saying, "You've got to be kidding me," and I waved him off. I took some Tylenol and drank a vitamin water for breakfast. I showered, dressed, barely able to lift up my feet to put on my scrubs, and drove to work, fighting the urge to put my head on the steering wheel. As soon as I walked into the hospital, I had to begin the fifty-five-patient rounding split among the three other residents. I was on shift for eighteen hours that day.

It seemed almost quaint that I once equated medical school with climbing Mount Everest. If anything, medical school was base camp. Neurosurgical residency was the attempt at the summit. Without oxygen. In the dark. While putting up your own ropes. While wearing a bathing suit. Yes, that's what neurosurgical residency was.

The show must go on. This is drilled into doctors and passed down through generations of doctors. However, this is one of the single biggest causes to physician burnout. When doctors are told to keep going, push emotions down, ignore our own illnesses, to keep working, don't show fatigue, we are unable to care for ourselves and, as a result, can't give optimal care to our patients. The longer I spent in my residency, the more I saw the signs of burnout all around me. Once again, my brain spun with the dread that I wasn't good enough, as good as I believed myself to be. That I wasn't strong enough. That I wasn't superhuman enough. As the first woman at Brown in thirteen years, I could not be the one to fail. That might make the administration say, "Look, see there? Women really aren't up to the task." And then it would be another thirteen years before another woman got a shot. Don't show vulnerability or weakness at work became a practice I carried home with me. *Don't let Alex or Mom and Dad or Jiji see you weak, Sheri. They won't understand what you're going through, and they can't help.* It was the saddest mantra in the world.

It was Dr. Cahill and the nurses who supported me, who allowed me space to go through what I needed to go through so I could come back renewed and focused. Some times were harder than others.

Sometimes there really were events that absolutely horrified me, and if I hadn't put a pin in that horror, I wouldn't have been able to treat my patient.

I had been up all night, the lone resident on-call for the fourth night in a row. Four nights in a row of being the skeleton crew. I hadn't showered, I was starving, and my feet felt like two blocks of immobile stone. I was well into my third year of neurosurgical residency, and I was wiped out. I had spent hours filling out death packets. As a Level 1 neurotrauma hospital, located off the busy Highway 95, we were the highest-level hospital in the state of Rhode Island. Neurotrauma patients arrived in droves even when it wasn't a warm holiday weekend. Shootings, spear-fishing trauma, car accidents, motorcycle accidents. Many times, patients arrived mostly dead or were coded, then pronounced dead. "Mostly dead" was not the same kind of "mostly dead" that Westley presented in *The Princess Bride*. Miracle Max could not bring these patients back with a magic chocolate-dipped pill.

I had thirteen ER consults and an external drain to place, but my hands were tired from the hours of paperwork. I'd stopped counting how many death packets I had completed after I reached fifty my intern year, but I had probably completed a dozen in the last few months on top of that number. There was so much death. And yet, it was the same amount of work to try to save them all.

As my pager went off for the thirtieth time that night, I put my head down on the desk, wishing it would swallow me up. I picked up the nearby phone with my head still down, and then I called the emergency room line. Dr. Stephens, the young ER resident I'd met our first Fourth of July, picked up. "Dr. Dewan," she said, "we have another live one for you. Young woman, early twenties, drunk driver, hit the Jersey barrier. She took a header through the windshield."

I ran down to the ER. The glass of the windshield scraped off her scalp. She had been scalped. Her scalp was gone, as was the top of her skull. Blood and glass and skin matted into her short, blond curls. What was there, in the open, was brain tissue and tiny little shards of glass from the windshield. It was like a gratuitous horror film that didn't even seem like it could be real—that's how vile it was. But I had to shut off the horror and get to work.

The chief resident was called and would meet us in the OR. First, I had to get the patient prepped for surgery by plucking glass from her wide-open cranium. This woman had been completely neurologically devastated at this point. It was gruesome. And then.

"Hi." The patient, whose brain was wide open and in my hand, looked up at me. She looked up at me and was talking to me.

Uh . . . "How are you feeling?" I asked her, making sure I was not imagining this.

"Oh," she said, a little confused, "my head hurts. I think my head hurts a lot." She sounded like someone ordering a cup of coffee.

Oh my god. Oh my god. "You're going to be okay; we're going to take care of you," I said.

"Yeah, you know, I think my head really hurts."

I plucked another piece of glass, trying to prep as much as I could to get this woman into surgery. "We're going to get you upstairs to surgery. We're going to take care of this."

"Okay. Yeah. Where am I right now?"

"You're at the hospital." *Her eyes are open and she's talking to me while my hands are in her brain. Don't freak out, Sheri. It's only like a scene from your least favorite movie in the entire world.*

"Oh. Did something happen to me? Why does my head hurt so much?"

"Your head hurts because you were in a car accident."

"Oh, a car accident. Ooooooooh. Uh-oh." Then she closed her eyes.

There had been a movie a few years earlier that Alex took me to see, along with some friends, when I was in graduate school. It was the sequel to *Silence of the Lambs*. The movie—*Hannibal*—features a scene in which Hannibal Lecter opens up Krendler's skull and cooks up a piece of his prefrontal cortex while Krendler is talking to him and Clarice. The movie terrified me. And now I was living that moment, without the eating and murder. This woman was awake and talking to me while I literally had my hands in her cranium.

Not now, Sheri, put a pin in it . . .

We rushed her up to surgery emergently for a craniotomy. As I ran with the stretcher and the surgical nurses, I held her brain with my hand. Once she was in the operating room, we had to irrigate the remaining shards out of the brain, very carefully and delicately. We had to shave down the edges of her skull and irrigate. She required a skin graft because so much scalp was missing, and we patched together whatever scalp we could. A plastic surgeon arrived to do the skin graft procedure.

I sent her to the ICU, scrubbed out, and was ready to curl up on a soiled stretcher lying in the middle of the hallway because I didn't have the energy to make it back to the residents' call room. That's when I was called in by the chief resident, who wanted to send me back into surgery with Dr. Cahill. I was so tired I wanted to die. In that moment, there was a passing thought of, *Well, if I keel over, at least I'll get to lie down.* That's how far gone I was.

When I trudged my way upstairs, the patient was ready for us in the OR, positioned face down on the operating table. The nurse prepped her lower spine, as we were to remove a four-centimeter spinal cord tumor wrapped around her lower nerves. Monitors blinked around us while nurses buzzed back and forth with the prep work, the anesthetists standing out of the way awaiting their cue. Dr. Cahill and I reviewed her scans on the computer then began the ceremonial process of dressing ourselves, the nurses assisting with the sterile gowning and gloving. The patient was draped and the site of the initial incision marked in purple ink.

Dr. Cahill and I worked silently, keeping our focus narrowed to the specific, meticulous task before us. This had to be done slowly. We worked in a concerted effort to perform the initial spinal opening, which alone took an hour. When the coverings of the spine were exposed, the microscope was wheeled in.

"Ah," Dr. Cahill said, his voice confident, ringing, "look, Sheri, here is the intradural portion of the tumor, just as I had expected! Am I good or what?" Yes, he was good, but I was not in the mood for offering congratulations. "That's how you operate," he continued.

"So," he said next, "how were your on-call responsibilities last night?"

Oh, you know, the usual. I spent the better part of an hour removing shards of glass from a woman's brain while she was awake, conscious, and talking to me, as if I was in an episode of The Twilight Zone.

Instead, I retorted, "It was a very long night, and I am in fact actively trying to erase it from my memory." We continued working, the silence punctuated by the machines and the occasional request from Dr. Cahill or his brief desire to chitchat.

"That's it, that's it, we are almost around the tumor," he bellowed, "and it's the swan song of this little bugger! Okay, send this to pathology, we are closing."

I looked at the clock; we had been in there seven hours exactly. Despite my comfy, worn-in clogs, my feet throbbed. My stomach rumbled, and my lower back ached.

"Dr. Dewan, you can close the dura, but I want it *tight tight tight*." He gave me a warning look. I knew what he wanted. No spinal fluid leaks, a sewn-tight dura with no holes. He wanted the Martha Stewart of sewing jobs.

I stepped up to the table and began closing, but, with the fatigue, my hands began to tremor. "I see your Parkinson's disease has kicked in, Dr. Dewan—you are off today."

I was not in the mood for his snide comments on a good day. Of course, I was off. I'd been up all night removing glass from someone's brain. "I just need some rest. I'll be on the mend. Don't worry, this dura will not leak." Nothing else mattered except this patient and my stitching. I got the job done.

I hadn't been ready to think about what I'd just experienced until after my shift ended and I got some good sleep. As horrible as the night had been, I kept returning to the image of holding the woman's brain in my hands while extracting glass shards and she was talking to me. I had done that. It was real. The accident had been terrible, and the patient was in bad shape, but setting that aside, holding a living brain was not an experience that most of the world's population would get to have, and it was incredible that I'd gotten to have it. Aside from sterilization and antibiotics and CT scans, the same principals I used were probably used by the Incans when they practiced trepanation.

I wanted to tell Alex about the woman and my whole experience, but when I started, he said, "Yikes, sounds gross."

What I really wanted to discuss was how I held two mutually exclusive or competing ideas in my head: How could I want to do this gruesome job? Why did I feel like I had to be there to try to save people if what I encountered was so viscerally tragic?

I knew my parents wouldn't want to hear about the way the brain had looked, studded with glass. Jiji would only tell me I wasn't normal . . . again. I had to deal with it in my own way.

I would learn to deal with every inhuman part of residency by putting aside the shock and trauma. I won't say that I got used to the fatigue part of my residency. It never felt natural for my body to not feel like my own. But I knew the steps, I knew how to get from Point A to D with a few stops in between. I wanted to be a highly evolved neurosurgeon; my body perfectly adapted for survival in my home terrain, much like a tiger's is for theirs. There was much I had to learn, especially with my nutrition.

An adult tiger can consume almost ninety pounds of meat in a single meal. It doesn't eat the entire kill at once, though; it will bury it and stay nearby, eating off it for days, going four or five days before it needs to kill again.[1] Since I wasn't a literal tiger, ninety pounds of meat would not work for me. Similarly, I learned that drinking a ton of water before a multi-hour surgery was not a good plan, as I discovered the first time I had to break scrub to pee. The same with coffee. Another of the residents recommended cranberry juice, which worked like a charm. The tartness revived me and provided enough sustenance to get me through multiple hours without overstimulating my bladder. I was grateful for all the tips. My system was evolving, and I was acquiring new instincts as my body accommodated. Taking care of my physicality was important, but I was still learning how to take care of my emotional life.

Habits were sometimes the only way to get through the tough emotional parts of the job. It's what I told myself one evening on the way to tell desperate parents their son didn't make it. In the waiting room, forty people, all family members, were nervous, crying, pacing, praying, and holding each other's hands. There I was, having to deliver the news that their teenage son, grandson, brother, and nephew was dead. Three different motorcycle accidents that day, all with the cyclists not wearing helmets, but his was by far the worst. His mother had been reluctant to leave his side when we wheeled him into surgery, and now he was gone. Eighteen years is nothing. It's a blink.

The brain was dead. Machines might keep the rest of the body alive artificially, until we stopped them. I had to ask this mother now what her wishes were, and if she would consider organ donation after brain death.

The particular shriek of the mother when I walked into the waiting room was nothing short of the most acute anguish. The sound echoed through me, and I fought to maintain composure.

"I'm so sorry," I repeated. I waited for the mother to be consoled, calmed enough so that I could set out the next steps, options for her to consider. She was inconsolable. I had yet to meet the parent who could remain stoic in a situation of this nature. A few hours earlier, they were all living a normal life. And then all they had was a shred of hope to cling to. And now that was gone.

Hope had carried me through my mother's aneurysm. Our family had been so lucky. How many times had this young man been lucky in his short life, riding his motorcycle without a helmet, and never having an accident?

After telling the family, I would wait for their decision on compassionate extubation. Directly after this, however, I had to meet Dr. Egan, a notoriously tough, glib, and aggressive (though brilliant) neurosurgeon in the OR for another surgery—another motorcycle accident—though this surgery wasn't as urgent; but first, I needed to take a moment for myself. I was shaken. I sat in the residents' office alone and tried to meditate, clear my thoughts, think of the surgery ahead.

I had to mentally prepare for all of that, plus the surgery. I called my parents to say hello, just to hear their voices. It was my way of finding my comfort, of putting myself back in a good space, and reorienting myself after being a part of another family's tragedy. After the call, I reminded myself that I had done everything that I could to save a life, that I couldn't save them all, but that there were other people I was going to save. Then, I drank a shot of cranberry juice and made my way to the next surgery.

I needed to get better at centering myself, so I started regular yoga and meditation. I learned the different variants, and I found that carving out even a little time each day for yoga and the quietness of mediation became my outlet for the stress and the burying of my emotions. Even if I didn't process everything every time, yoga and meditation made me feel better and helped me let go of some of that perpetual anxiety. In a perfect world, I would have done it every day, twice a day, but sneaking in small sections whenever I could made a big difference in being able to cope. The moments were few, but when it was all I had, those moments became tiny miracles in my day. It helped me, and in turn, it helped my patients. Yoga also helped me not dwell on the traumas once I came home. I couldn't dump it all on Alex, but also, I wouldn't resent him for not being able to listen to every single story and understand it in the same way I did.

You might not burn out, but if you don't process the traumas you experience, you can damage the relationships around you. Passion has to be the polestar, but unprocessed trauma can derail you from your dreams even if you have the world's greatest map and a stellar support system. The processing of the trauma will have to come from you. If you're fortunate and can use your closest supporters to help you process, then you have additional help. But there will be those times you have to postpone that processing and just survive the moment.

I like to think that part of putting a pin in it is like "driving through the danger." I learned this idea early on in my childhood while living in Saudi Arabia. We had to leave the country every six months to avoid being eligible for citizenship. That meant my parents planned wonderful trips for us to places near Saudi Arabia that we wouldn't otherwise have gotten to see for years, if at all. One of these trips coincided with the height of Tut-Mania, the 1970s tour of *The Treasures of Tutankhamun* (which came to Chicago right when we weren't there). Jiji was all in with her Tut-Mania, and we both were enthralled with Egyptology as a result. We were at the heights of ecstasy when our parents announced the trip to Egypt.

"Finally!" I shouted.

"Can I get a mattock?" Jiji asked. She was ready to dig up her own mummified pharaoh.

My mother sent us to the bookcase instead, where we pulled out books on Egypt and the pharaohs. "You can dig in these," our mother said. "And then you can lead the way and be our tour guides."

The planning of the trip and our research solidified the obsession. We made up stories and realities about Tut, about the pharaohs, and we imagined ourselves exploring tombs and making mummies. (Ironically, ancient Egyptians didn't think the brain was important, which was why it was scrambled or liquefied, pulled out through the nose, and not stored in a Coptic jar.)[2] One night, as we slept in our bunk beds, I awoke to Jiji's voice, muttering, "King Tut was the pharaoh of the eighteenth dynasty, reigned during the New Kingdom . . . " then something more about dates. She was asleep. She was reciting the introduction to one of our new books by one of the Tut/Egyptology authors with three initials in his name (though I'm the weird one). During this time, I regularly had to wake her up in the middle of sleeptalking about King Tut. "You're keeping me up!" I'd call down to her bottom bunk.

"No, I wasn't!"

"Yes, you were! Again!"

We were beyond excited when the date of our trip came. We would be going to Tut's tomb, and we also were set to go to the Great Pyramid, which wasn't always open.

"Be careful, though," one of our guides warned us. Despite our avid research, Jiji and I would not be the sole designated guides for our trip; my parents hired professional local guides, and they warned us, "Do not go to the tombs at dusk. Many robberies at that time of day, sometimes more than robberies, worse than robberies. Only go during the day."

The daytime was hot, though. Very hot. The temperature hovered at ninety-nine degrees, and it was dusty. Coming from Saudi Arabia, a neighboring country, I thought I'd be used to the heat. And isn't Cairo on the coast?

Well. Cairo is about a three-hour drive to the coast. It's on the Nile, but that only makes it cooler than the Eastern Desert. The heat in Cairo was more stifling than Dhahran, as if the air came into our lungs but never quite expired out. Also, unlike Dhahran, where I always felt safe, there was an undercurrent of danger everywhere we went—robbers at the tombs or in the city streets, not to mention mummy curses.

The day we went to one of the pyramids with the local guide, we took a car, and he warned us, "Do not open the windows under any circumstances." Air conditioning in the car, however, was limited at that time. We had some beat-up old beige car, the color of a blast of sand, and as our driver navigated the slow, choking traffic of Cairo, we gagged and choked on the exhaust fumes the car was expelling directly into the air vents. The car might have been a mummy's curse. The heat, the fumes, the suffocating air of the back seat of that dingy car, the pestilence the car was belching, it was too much. It was the eleventh plague of Egypt. We opened the back window. We stopped for traffic, then started up again, making our way to the main hub of town. We slowed again, then the beige bane came to a stop. There was a man walking along the side of the road, looking at cars. I had just enough time to see something wrapped around his arm before all of a sudden, his arm reached into our car window, directly toward my father's face. Wrapped around his arm was a cobra.

The man had one hand grasped at the cobra's tail, his other grasping the snake's neck so that its mouth was forced open, wide. He yelled in Arabic, then in English, for my father to give him money or he would throw the cobra into the car. We lurched forward as the car surged into traffic, and with a *thunk*, the snake and the arm were ejected from the window. The beige jalopy moved as fast as it could go.

"Close the window!" our guide yelled. Eyes wide, we complied. This was not Dhahran, indeed.

I had up until then understood that there were undercurrents of danger throughout the world, but I had been sheltered from them for most of my life. Even when we traveled, places like Macau and Hong Kong, we were not exposed to the unsafe.

We made it to the pyramid that day, and Jiji and I scampered over the ancient stones, soaking up every second. We weren't affected by the heat at all, not while we were exploring. We listened to everything the guide told us about the pharaoh, about how the slaves might have carried up the stones (though new evidence since has offered up other theories). I imagined coming back as an adult, digging through rock and sand, dusting off etched hieroglyphics to reveal a three-thousand-year-old story. The point was that despite the danger, we had a wonderful day. Our guide took special care of us and stretched out history for my hand to touch. We put ourselves in a dangerous situation by ignoring advice and taking a risk. But once we were elbow deep in risk, there were only two ways things could turn out: with a loss, or with a bold move to drive through the danger. That became something of a family mantra. Whether the dangers were self-inflicted or not, sometimes you have to be prepared to react and then process, deduce lessons, and move on.

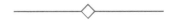

It takes guts to make tough goals, and the road to success is hard. Even with all the planning, sometimes you have to do what you know is risky. If it's worth doing, it's worth the risk. (Though always follow the advice of your Egyptian guides.) I had to drive through the danger of my residency to have the life I always wanted: being in the operating room on my own terms. Choosing neurosurgery meant that there would be glass in brains, there would be brains coming out of noses, there would be cases that would break my heart. I had to be able to deal with that, acknowledge how much a patient loss hurt, and sit with it. Then, I had to remind myself that I had done everything that was in my power, as I did every time, and not punish myself if a patient was beyond saving.

Putting a pin in your emotions can't be a permanent state. Yes, you drive through the danger, get to a safe place, and then you can process and take stock of the experience. From there, you find a way forward. From there, you recenter yourself, take off some of the load through meditation or being with people who love and support you, whatever works best for you to stay on your path.

7

———

Remind Yourself What's Temporary

Temporary—it's an important word.

I used it to get me through my mother's therapy sessions, her early incapacitation and inability to care for herself. Eventually, we did all get past The Aneurysm. The Great Despair. The Family Tragedy. My mother wasn't suddenly recovered and back to her old self, but we found—and were happy with—this new version of my mom brought back from not only death but severe debilitation. We, of course, were lucky. The thing is, traumas don't always go away. That's why it's important to cling to small victories, to make new goals, and to take things bite-size, when it all seems too much.

Temporary is also an important concept to remember when dealing with stress from tasks that seem insurmountable. Tasks that you know you have to take on in order to have the life you want. There will be heavy lifting, and at times, there's no way around it. That's when you have to drive *through* the danger. That's why you have to keep reminding yourself to be passionate and that your moonshot goal is absolutely worth the usually temporary trials and tribulations.

This is a separate component from dealing with trauma, which isn't always temporary—the loss of a loved one is an extreme example. I couldn't tell the mother of the eighteen-year-old motorcyclist that the pain from the loss of her son is temporary. Her grief may change and evolve, and there may be some mothers who might channel that grief into some kind of action, which is a wholly personal decision. But most of us have had the moments where you cling to the knowledge that the pain will pass—childbirth is an obvious example, as is potty training a child or puppy.

Anyone who has waited until the last minute to finish a term paper knows this feeling acutely. Though there can be deep cuts, deep pains that feel like they will last forever, they heal over so well that you don't feel the suffering anymore. You might never forget the memory of it, but the pain will dissipate, and the end result makes the trial worth it.

———◇———

I had told myself: "Medical school is temporary."

I regularly reminded myself: "Residency is temporary."

I would learn acutely: "Pregnancy is temporary."

Yes, in my fifth year of residency, and at the age of thirty-one, I got pregnant with my first daughter. Alex had been ready for this since our wedding, much earlier than I was, and I certainly couldn't have taken a break any time earlier during my residency to have a baby. By this time, though, I was ready to be a mom and didn't want to push it off for another two or three years.

We planned to name our daughter Amara, after my grandfather, Amar Narayan Agarwal, who was a gilded figure my entire life, even though he was killed in an Indian Airlines plane crash just before I was born. He was a well-known economics professor at the University of Allahabad before he helped found Jawaharlal Nehru University. He published several books on economic policy and development in India, and ultimately, one of his textbooks became the national textbook for all the schools in India. He branched out, giving lectures all over the world, including frequent lectures at Stanford and University of Michigan, Ann Arbor. Just before his plane went down, he was tapped to be the Indian ambassador to Rhodesia, present-day Zimbabwe.

Alex and I flew back to Illinois to tell my parents the news; my mother would be around to see my child born, and she was now well enough to fully enjoy being a grandmother. She and my father even arranged to come out for Amara's birth and my mom would stay with us for the first six weeks to help us take care of the new baby. All those years ago, while I awaited my mother's recovery during those long days in the ICU, I had wished for this very moment.

"Okay," my mom said, wiping her eyes upon hearing the news, "so are you staying healthy? You're not getting fatigued at work, are you? What about nutrition—are you taking prenatal vitamins?"

I laughed and said everything was fine, that it was all normal. Every time we talked over the phone for the rest of my pregnancy, my mom was so concerned with my health and wanting to make sure I wasn't pushing myself to exhaustion. "It's not just about *your* health, either," she said.

There were a few secrets I had to keep. I didn't tell her about the overnight calls I had to take. I didn't tell her about the thirty-hour shifts that continued through my pregnancy.

At work, it was time to share the news of my pregnancy with my colleagues. This did not go over as hoped. "Great, and who's going to be stuck with all your call while you're out on maternity leave?" one of the residents asked.

There was no question I would make up the call. My plan was to take all the call in the weeks leading up to my maternity leave, which would be six weeks long. Fortunately, there were a couple of residents on my side, or at least, a couple who were happy to work out a solution. And I took all my six weeks' worth of call before my delivery. There was no way I wanted to make that up on the back end, not when I would have a baby to take care of. I would be taking call every few nights. If fatigue was bad during the residency before I was pregnant, add to that the fatigue from growing a person and taking extra overnight shifts.

I was supposed to be happy—and I was happy. But I was also frustrated at the reaction.

I overheard one conversation in the hallways, between two of the attendings. "Doesn't she know that she shouldn't get pregnant? There is no such thing as a good neurosurgeon and a good mother—didn't she know that?"

Um, what?

These were doctors who knew me, who knew my work. I was a senior resident. Suddenly, they were doubting me, my judgment, what I was capable of doing. I understand the anxiety to an extent. Being someone who was regularly sent to the bookshelves, I knew how to do my research. One statistic tells that over 40 percent of qualified, professional women leave their careers when they have children.[1]

Part of the problem, in any career, can be the lack of assistance for working moms. A quarter of moms return to work within two weeks of giving birth because they can't take the pay cut of full maternity leave, or their employers will fill their positions with someone else. Plenty of other women would just rather stay home with their kids and have the privilege of not needing to work. Some new mothers imagine taking only a year or two off, then find it difficult to reintegrate into the workplace or even to find a job. Sometimes the year or two turns into a decade. These are even women with advanced degrees. Employers often—obliquely—cite this phenomenon as the reason to not pay women a wage equivalent to what men would make.[2]

Their thought process often goes that while women are qualified, if they leave to have a kid, they have to train someone else to take her place, ultimately costing them time and money. This idea has been discussed in media, news, and journal articles, and I have nothing new to add to the discussion.

What I did have was my certainty that I was born to be a neurosurgeon and had spent my entire life building toward that goal. I also knew I wanted to be a mother. I would love my children, I already knew, but I was always going to be a neurosurgeon. I was going to bet on myself; I could be a neurosurgeon and a mother. It would be difficult, that I already knew. I would be asking a lot from Alex, but it was a discussion we had, one we'd been having since before I went into medical school.

Two weeks after I announced my pregnancy, fellow doctors were still doling out . . . I don't know if I can call it advice. Ominous warnings?

On one day, it was Dr. Evans, the neurosurgeon with several children, ranging in age from mid-teens to early twenties. "They say having children is hard; having children as a resident is even harder!"

You don't say?

While scrubbing out of a craniotomy a few days later, the assisting resident said to me, "You know Sheri, what they say is true. There really is no such thing as a good neurosurgeon and good father. They say that about mothers too, you know."

I don't know what they expected me to do about this. I was already pregnant. I had wanted to become pregnant. Were they challenging me to quit? Were these comments effectively a version of putting down their names in an office pool of when Sheri would leave the field?

Upset again, I researched online that night when I went home and found a study discussing neurosurgery attrition rates for the previous decade. Attrition during or just after residency for neurosurgeons is actually quite low. Over three-quarters obtained board certification, with men at slightly higher rates than women, though the study didn't cite the causes for attrition. Graduates of higher institutions had somewhat higher attrition rates than public medical schools, which probably spoke more to factors relating to medical school debt and being able to go into practice than any other cause, though the study didn't separate women from men in that aspect.[3]

Alex came up to me from behind my shoulder. "Whatcha reading?" He leaned in closer to the screen. "Sheri, tell me you are not really worried about this."

"No, of course I'm not worried. I just—all I'm hearing from the residents and attendings is that it can't be done."

I was worried, though. Was it the right decision to even think about having a child during my residency? Could a woman be a neurosurgeon and a mother?

Alex rubbed my shoulders. "But you don't believe it can't be done. I certainly don't believe it can't be done. I mean, people have kids and are neurosurgeons. It is actually done. And you can do anything you put your mind to, ergo . . . "

I laughed.

"You're a great neurosurgeon. At least that's the rumor about town." I'd had my head down, and he leaned forward to look me in the eye. "And I know that you will be a great mom. Plus, you got me, so how could we not totally rock this thing? These fools are saying I can't be a killer neurosurgeon spouse? Give me a break!"

How lucky I was to have Alex. And here was the thing: all the neurosurgeon spouses I had met thus far, and all that I have known since, they have all been tough as nails. They knew the load they were taking on. They could handle spending life alone a lot of the time. They could run a household and a family, taking care of what needed to get done, many of them while holding down jobs of their own.

Alex's experience as an expectant father was entirely different. Still a postdoctoral fellow, his colleagues and professors at Brown were ecstatic for us. They planned two baby showers, one thrown for me by his boss, and the other thrown by his coworkers. They were there to give me much-needed advice. I had no idea how to raise a baby. What do you do? What do you feed them? How do you feed them? How do you take their temperature? Alex's advisor was a mother herself. She took the time to type up long lists of advice in lengthy emails with such information as what bath temperature to use, how to feed and keep a log, how to keep track of everything. Her input was invaluable for me. I was so grateful, but it only highlighted the disparity in reactions from my own colleagues.

As my baby grew, kicked, and squirmed, the work continued. Where I did receive support? The hospital staff and other patients. The nurses, especially the cadre of Portuguese nurses, office assistants, and orderlies, were the most enthusiastic supporters outside of my family. They were the people who knitted me baby blankets and booties and little hats with soft yarn. One of them told me that it was custom—no, the rule—if a pregnant woman wanted anything, especially sweets, they were supposed to be given it. It's a sign of good luck. I couldn't walk past the nurses' station without somebody offering me a freshly homemade Portuguese cookie. They would also rub my back in the operating room after a long case.

Then, as I began to show, suddenly, it was as if patients saw me in a different light. I became human to them. I wasn't just a doctor, surgeon, or neurosurgeon; my humanity grew as my belly grew. The support I received from them, the adoring stares, the sincere congratulations, all of these were daily gifts, individuals coming to my aid when I needed them most.

Neurosurgery and motherhood were from then on inextricably bound for me. I felt my baby's first kicks while I was operating—for the first time feeling new life as I was working to save a life. That was a feeling that is hard to compare to any other feeling. There were times, though, when I had to fight not to let my pregnancy affect my performance.

I was on my way to perform a craniotomy to remove a brain tumor with Dr. Evans that morning. The patient was a sharp, diligent, and astute attorney from a prominent law firm in Boston. She had been in court during a legal proceeding and had a grand mal seizure with loss of consciousness. Rushed to the hospital, a brain tumor was revealed, located in her right frontal lobe, pushing on the ventricles, or water drainage system of the brain. She wanted to fight this. Adamant to have the best possible outcome, she was prepared to have surgery immediately. I wanted to give her the best outcome I could, remove the tumor as safely possible, and give her hope. I also wanted to keep from vomiting due to morning sickness.

The patient was prepped and draped in a field of blue, her hair shaved and medicalized, her body without any visible signs of life from my side of the drape. I was in my second trimester, belly now a firm, round ball that pushed up against the operating room table, causing a distance between me and the patient. I wished for longer arms. I injected local anesthetic into her subcutaneous scalp layers, then made my cut with the scalpel. Bleeding was stopped with a cautery instrument. I made the incision down to the bone, exposing the shiny skull. Then, Shannon, the scrub nurse, brought in the navigation equipment—the proverbial GPS system for the brain. It was like a wand that could locate and map the tumor, allowing for smaller incisions, smaller craniotomies. The goal is to minimize the opening of the skull and minimize the exposure of the brain. I mapped her craniotomy, then removed the small, bony flap using the high-speed drill.

Then, Dr. Evans entered the room, looking over my work. "I have to say, that is quite a nice craniotomy, no excessive bleeding, yes that is good. Kill that tumor, Dewan, just kill it."

He chatted leisurely with the OR staff about his latest vacation to the Greek Islands. As he was discussing all the risks and benefits of group yachting versus private vessel cruising, I opened the dura and looked at her pulsating frontal lobe.

"Bring in the microscope, lights off in the room," I ordered.

The tumor was pink and fleshy, tentacles reaching into her eloquent brain structures. I found a ragged border around the tumor and began the resection. The tumor had a clear boundary and was easily resecting with no significant bleeding. This was going well. I sent the first specimen to the pathologist and held my breath for a moment.

Just then, a wave of nausea came over me. It hit like a tsunami, and I nearly toppled over. I choked and gagged. I had to stay composed. I could not let Dr. Evans see any sign of weakness in me. I could not let my pregnancy affect my performance. I started to sweat.

Dr. Evans continued his tale with fervor to an audience of nurses. "And then, I said to my wife, 'This is the life, really it is. Let's retire here!' Hey, Dewan—what's going on over there?"

What do you think is going on? I'm hunched over a brain about to vomit. I'm six months pregnant. "Just making my way around this tumor," I said. "It's almost out."

"Why don't I scrub in and help you out?" he said.

No, no, no. I got this, just let me take a deep breath. One deep breath. I inhaled and exhaled, trying to fight the nausea as I fought my patient's brain tumor. I refocused my energies.

I will this away. I no longer need to vomit. I do not need to vomit. I cannot vomit. I will not vomit. This is ridiculous, I'm in the middle of a craniotomy. The tumor is almost out. I pushed away the notion of scrubbing out, or vomiting in my mask, or any such horror. I concentrated on the task at hand.

My mind began to trick my body.

"It's out, the tumor is out," I said to the anesthesiologist. "We are going to start closing."

"I'll go update the patient's family," Dr. Evans said, exiting the operating room.

Breathing a small sigh of relief, I began reapproximating the dura.

Shannon leaned close to me, ensuring no one else in the room could hear. "You almost didn't make it," she whispered in her thick East Coast accent. "You are doing so well, by the way. I don't know how you managed to do this job pregnant." She smiled and, above her surgical mask, the lines around her crystal green eyes deepened. Shannon had been a neurosurgery scrub nurse for over twenty-five years and had seen countless residents come and go. Her stories were the woven fabric of the hospital quilt, each piece of patchwork memorialized with each graduating resident.

"I can't imagine any other reality," I said. "This is my job. This is my office." I shook off the last of my wooziness, stabilizing myself by leaning my belly against the table.

She nodded. "Sher, someday you will have your own schedule and your own life. You will choose when to operate, what time, what day. But for now, you have *this.*"

This was the indentured servitude of residency. Having no control over when you slept, ate, showered, studied, no semblance of free time. Knowing that a light existed at the end of a very long and arduous tunnel made the difference. Seven years was a long time for servitude, especially when that time span entailed my early thirties. But now, at least, I was well past the halfway point.

A few days later, while I was scheduling my call schedule, taking on more of what I would have to miss during my six weeks of maternity leave, one of the senior residents made a snarky comment about my pregnancy. "Dewan, are you smuggling basketballs into the call room again?" One of the residents smirked and cocked an eyebrow.

It was the persecution of pregnancy. My growing belly might as well have been stamped with a scarlet "P" for all to see and judge. One would have thought I'd committed a crime, killed someone, made some atrocious medical error. Was there this expectation that all neurosurgeons were expected to live, breathe, and eat neurosurgery without having any semblance of a normal existence? Was it really about taking off six weeks of time?

In fact, the last resident who had required six weeks off was a male. He broke his leg skiing.

Then I heard Dr. Cahill at my side. "Sheri, can I borrow you for a minute?"

He walked with me down the hallway, then rounded the corner. He leaned in close. "You do what you need to do for you and your child. Do not pay any attention to the rest." He looked at me like a father would. I was so grateful to him. He rarely let his humanity show on full display; it was hard for a seasoned neurosurgeon to do. But I realized just how much humanity he had.

The truth is that I began to feel disabled as I became more pregnant, a person who has no oxygen to climb stairs or walk through a parking lot. Between the weight and blood volume increase, I felt like a waddling mass. I fantasized about living outside my body.

I worked up until my water broke. I was due between Christmas and New Year's, and I'd had it in my head that Christmas would be it. However, Christmas came and went. My parents had flown out to celebrate with us, and also to be present—and available to help—once our baby was born. Two days after Christmas, I woke up and was over being pregnant. I had broken out into a Pruritic Urticarial Papules and Plaques of Pregnancy (PUPPP) rash, which is the opposite of a soft and cuddly and wet-nosed pup. About one out of every 250 pregnant women contract this horrible and vile rash of raised red bumps and blotches, which often starts on the belly but frequently spreads to the extremities, lasting sometimes for weeks, and is one of the many things not welcomed when you're swollen, fatigued, sore, and hormonal. My body itched all the time, and I couldn't put hydrocortisone on it. The only thing that works is Benadryl, and when you're pregnant, you don't want to take Benadryl because it affects the baby's mentation and sensory system.

Please let my water break, please let my water break. I said it like a new mantra as I rolled myself out of bed and took a cool shower to relieve the persistent burning itch of what were basically hives. Then, I put on the loosest-fitting clothes I had before sitting on the couch. All day, everyone was staring at me—Alex, my parents—waiting for the baby to come out. Then, at 5:00 p.m., my water broke. Right there.

The Women and Infants Hospital of Rhode Island was close and everything went smoothly. The only catch was that at the same time, there was an outbreak of swine flu. Alex was the only person allowed in the delivery room, and only one person at a time would be able to visit. My Portuguese staff, all eager to pop by to see the new baby, would have to wait. Even hospital staff couldn't congregate here. My parents would only be able to come one at a time, but they drove with us and sat in the waiting room.

And then, it was time. But then it wasn't. Or rather, it was time for thirty hours. Then, when she finally came out, she didn't make a sound. Her APGARs were low. But after one whack on her bottom from the obstetrician, she started screaming her lungs out. That's when I knew I had a healthy girl. The nurse handed my baby girl to me wrapped up in lined baby blankets. I couldn't believe that something so beautiful and perfect had come from my body.

"Hello, Amara."

All of the frustrations over the months of my pregnancy were flushed away as I held her. A couple of hours later, my mom was allowed into the room with us so she could meet Amara. When my mother came in the room, teary-eyed, to meet her first grandchild, if it was possible, my heart filled even more than it had the moment Amara was born.

"There she is!" my mom said, reaching out and taking Amara in her arms.

My mother couldn't hike the Annapurna's now, but she was here, she was holding my daughter, she had lived and thrived and now held her granddaughter nearly ten years after she had almost died.

"Mom," I said, wiping a tear from my cheek. She looked at me and nodded.

"Beautiful Amara," she said, her father's name rolling from her lips. She leaned down to touch her forehead to Amara's little capped and pink forehead.

I wasn't natural at knowing all the ins and outs of being a new parent, and that's where my mom led the charge. However, it turned out that I was a natural at one particular aspect of being a new parent: midnight feedings. Amara would cry to be fed, and it was just like another page coming in from a call shift. I would get up, feed Amara, rock her back to sleep, and then go back to sleep myself. It was a breeze. Poor Alex had a much more difficult time adjusting to interrupted sleep.

The six weeks of my maternity leave flew by. And my mother couldn't live with us permanently. She still had her life back in Illinois, and my dad was alone at home; she wanted to get back to him. After a long search, Alex and I found a great nanny to be the daily caregiver for Amara, without whom Alex and I would have been totally lost.

Though I was sad to say goodbye to my mom and to leave Amara during the day, the truth was that I was excited to get back to work. I missed the OR. I missed the patients, scrubbing in for surgery, doing whatever I could to fix them.

Giving birth and then taking care of a newborn and going back to work was the single hardest thing I have ever done. I thought of all the women all over the world, women in India who give birth in the fields, cut the umbilical cord with a reed, and then go right back to work—what women are capable of is truly amazing. Especially all of the single mothers who have to be everything: mother, father, breadwinner, caretaker, nurturer. I had a friend who was a single mom, and though I was always in awe of what she was able to do, becoming a working mom made me realize the sheer immensity of that task. If they're all doing it, I can too.

Shannon, the scrub nurse who promised me one day would be different and my schedule would be my own, was absolutely right. Though my trials of residency were not yet over, each of them was a temporary roadblock. Fortunately, keeping sight of my moonshot goal and staying passionate would get me through every single one.

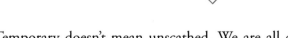

Temporary doesn't mean unscathed. We are all changed and shaped by our experiences—some for the better, sometimes for the worse. The key is to take advantage of what agency we have over our paths. Returning to the theme of determination and the use of the word grit: grit works best when applied to what you know will be a temporary hard patch. While I wish my pregnancy with Amara would have been easier, filled with relaxation and the ability to wallow in all the love to come, that's not the experience I was given. That's okay. I couldn't control my rash or my colleagues' reactions, but I could control how much it got me down. I had to rely on my determination, my passion, and my knowledge that I was making the choices in my life that I wanted to make.

That's what you have to do: cling to the times you get to make your own choices, and in the times when you can't, when you have to drive through danger and put a pin in everything else, remind yourself that there are great things waiting for you on the other end. But be realistic, though. Going through one tough spot doesn't mean that everything else will be easy. Take advantage of the tools and people you have to help you through whatever comes next.

8

Be All In

Speaking of roadblocks . . .

There are times when simple determination and faith in the *temporary* will not suffice, when you're at the precipice of giving up on your dream. This is the time when a decision is necessary, when you have to tell yourself that you are on this path no matter what or decide that it's time to call it all off.

This is a chapter about what to do when you reach the *nadir*, the lowest of lows, the great potential derailment of your dream, the scrapped launch of your moonshot, and how to keep going, despite it all.

At least, here's my story.

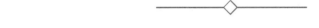

My first pregnancy didn't go over well with my fellow residents and attendings, but in my mind, I had proven that I could handle motherhood and neurosurgery. I guess I assumed better, because my second pregnancy really sent them into a tailspin.

I got pregnant a year later—on purpose. I wanted to have my children close together, and Alex and I figured since we had a great nanny and everything had worked out so well the first time, it was an ideal time to go ahead and raise two children who would be very close in age and development. We were going to be having another girl—Mia.

As I had before, I would be taking maternity leave again, frontloading all my twenty-four-hour call. I heard the comments behind my back, which was unnecessary since many of my colleagues also addressed their derision directly toward me.

"Do you really think you're going to come back to this after having *two* kids?" one colleague said.

I took a deep breath and tried to keep even tempered, despite the hormones and frustration coursing through me. "Yes. Yes, I do. I did it once, so I know I can do it again."

"Yeah," he said, "but two kids? I'm just saying, a lot of female residents who have kids don't come back after maternity leave. And that's not even in neurosurgery."

I wanted to say that maybe the ones who don't come back are the ones who get no support from colleagues, but I put on what was probably a dismissive smile and said, "Well, I can't speak for any other doctor, but this is what I'm doing."

Not that there weren't additional difficulties that pregnancy added on.

I had finally made it through the weeks of morning sickness, but I had to make sure I stayed hydrated and got enough chances to rest. After rounding on twenty-five patients, I was physically exhausted and sat down for a little break. My phone rang, and it was Dr. Stephens down in the ER. "Sheri? I think you really need to see this lady. They found her living in squalor, they said she was a hoarder, and her house was just full to the top with junk. She hasn't showered in probably over a year, and well . . . she has something growing out of her head."

Growing out of her head? Okay, likely clinical scenarios: maybe a large brain tumor that may have eroded through the brain cortices, into the skull, possible infection, but the description offered by Dr. Stephens, and her seeking consultation from me . . . I was trepidatious as I pushed myself out of the chair, finished my water, and walked down to the ER.

The patient was located in one of the small rooms off to the side, not in the trauma pod, but in one of the two pods for the less acute patients. When I walked into the room, it was as if I was hit by a tsunami of odor: a combination of garbage and feces, like the dirty Indian bathrooms of my childhood vacations with my parents. I recalled the movie *Trainspotting* when Ewan McGregor's character goes into "the worst toilet in Scotland." Now imagine that it is actually a porta potty, in a derelict region of a large city, and it hasn't been cleaned in months. That is something of the quality of this smell. Suddenly, my morning sickness didn't feel quite like a thing of the past.

In the bed lay a cachectic (someone whose muscles have wasted away), decrepit woman with dirty blonde hair. Reviewing her MRI scan, I found she did have an invasive tumor, something called a meningioma, which can erode from the brain cortices and, if left unchecked, can move further into the skull and cause hyperostosis, which is excessive growth of bony tissue. If left unchecked over time, it could develop into a large growth over the scalp. This patient's meningioma had apparently eroded through the skull and was fungating outside the head.

There was nobody in the room with her. I couldn't blame them, but my heart hurt for this pitiful woman. I introduced myself, and keeping her eyes down, she said, "I don't want to be here."

What I wanted to say was, "Neither do I," but I reminded myself that my job was to take care of patients. I put on gloves and walked over to her, gasping to maintain my composure. The smell was on an entirely different level, and the closer I got, the worse it was. The nausea crept in. If only I had Vicks VapoRub with me now.

I began my examination through the matted hair, where the tumor was eroding, and I noticed small, squiggly creatures, realizing for the first time that she had maggots in her hair. As I held the first maggot in my gloved hand, I couldn't contain it anymore. I jumped up, ripped off my gloves, and ran into the adjoining room, mercifully empty, and vomited into the trashcan.

I took a moment to compose myself. I couldn't believe this was a living, breathing individual with maggots in her hair, coming into the hospital with a fungating tumor, in the United States of America. This was something you'd see in a developing country without access to medical care. It shouldn't be happening in the US. Here in Rhode Island. And she was not a homeless woman. But there was no one looking out for her, advocating for her care.

I knew I had to go back in. Once I calmed down, I pumped some hand sanitizer into my hand and rubbed it under my nose. This time, I grabbed a mask and gown to protect myself from any infectious process, and double gloved. I pulled out the maggots. I had to shave her hair around the growth of the tumor because her hair was so matted, and then I sent her to be prepped for surgery. She had to be cleansed, and it was left to the nurses to scrub the remaining hair. She was admitted to the ICU, and the plastic surgeons joined me there for a consult. Once we got her to surgery, I would remove the tumor, and the area would be debrided with a large scalp flap that would have to be rotated by the plastic surgery team.

News of the "maggot lady" spread through our department, and the other residents were both fascinated by the story and grateful they were spared having to take care of her. For a few, the fact that I had been the one to handle this patient (the most horrific sight I still to this day have ever seen in a patient), while pregnant, assuaged some of their concerns about my willingness to do the job. I was committed, and so they let up.

There was one attending, though, who took particular exception to my condition: Dr. Egan—the brilliant but tough, insincere, and combative neurosurgeon who enjoyed making his residents squirm. Whenever I was within earshot, he would make comments such as, "I guess not everyone has the same level of dedication to their field," or when assisting on a surgery, he would casually drop in the chestnut, "Being a neurosurgeon is a commitment some people just aren't willing to see through, I guess."

It wasn't even that there was a terrible inconvenience against this man. He would not be the one to cover my call. He wasn't even doing the scheduling. I think he had a morbid desire to see me fail. Maybe desire isn't the right word—fascination, maybe. Like someone who watches a horrible accident with excitement. My pregnancy was a personal affront to him and everything he worked for.

To stress the point again, it is difficult to be a neurosurgeon regardless of gender. It would be impossible without a network of support. Spouses of neurosurgeons have a Herculean task that is sometimes akin to being a single parent. It's almost like a military partnership, each of us generals on different fronts. We couldn't win the war without each other, but we have to be able to work independently in order to get the job done. Alex and I wanted the same things and were supportive of each other's careers, and we would do what it took to have the life we wanted. I could face down the passive aggression (sometimes not so passive) knowing that I was coming home to Alex every night—or every morning after a twenty-four-hour call.

But as with a few other careers, women in neurosurgery are so often told they can't do it, that they don't belong, that they just aren't neurosurgeons. There is a built-in expectation of failure that goes beyond what men in neurosurgery face. Maybe not every woman is cut out to be a neurosurgeon, but certainly many men don't make it, either (it was a male resident who had left during my tenure). There is nothing physically that makes men more apt to the tasks of neurosurgery than women. The difference, it seems to me, is in expectations. Some people see a woman and think *she can't.* For a woman to succeed, there is the expectation that she will have to become genderless. Hard to be genderless with a full pregnant belly. Now that I was pregnant (for the second time), the thinking apparently went, I would or should (or wanted to) stay at home. Yet no one I encountered talked about men in neurosurgery this way.

I would have to prove them wrong, and not simply because I wanted to put these particular naysayers in their place (although that would be a bonus). I had spent my life preparing for this, and nearly the last decade training to become a neurosurgeon.

I couldn't control how I was treated, but I could deal with it. Unfortunately, ingrained misogyny is not the only hazard of being a neurosurgeon. Especially not for a pregnant woman working on-call with trauma patients who are uncooperative and intoxicated.

Six months pregnant with Mia, I had a patient come in drunk and violent, and with a spinal fracture. I was attempting to fixate her spine in an external device called a halo, a somewhat medieval metal ring with several screws surrounding the skull, affixed to a vest with rods. When I tried to put her in the halo to keep her steady, she punched me in the belly. Mia kicked and squirmed, and the nurse told me to immediately go get checked, and despite the initial scares, fortunately, everything was fine. However, even after that, I didn't want to shy away from the work, to give anyone leverage to say, "Look, pregnant women can't handle the work."

Oh, I would handle it, I told myself. It was a matter of rolling up my sleeves.

Except. There was finally the time I almost was no longer able to handle it.

A month after the aggressive woman punched my pregnant belly, I was openly berated. It was Monday morning Grand Rounds (pimping) conference, the cross between diagnosing and debugging a case that did not have a favorable outcome the previous week. It was also more than a little bit of hazing, and we were simultaneously interviewing the candidates for the next cycle of residency. We were on our third round of twenty young and eager medical students. Somewhere in the auditorium that day was possibly another me, the one neurosurgical candidate who would be selected for Brown's residency program. The candidates stood at the back of the amphitheater, leaning against the wall, digesting the presented talks and cases, absorbing what life would be like for the next seven years.

If the future candidate was in the room that day, they were a witness to my own hazing.

It seemed as my abdomen grew and hardened, so did the anger of the attending who had made most of the snide remarks during my pregnancy—Dr. Egan. The passive aggressive comments swelled into public displays of anger at the week's Grand Rounds.

I was not actually presenting that day; it was someone else's case. I had been operating the majority of the night. A motorcyclist, riding without a helmet, had arrived with an epidural hematoma—an arterial blood clot that compresses the surface of the brain, causing the brain tissues to shift. If not dealt with promptly, this condition can be fatal. I was the resident on-call, as I was always on-call in the months leading up to delivery, when the patient was brought to the trauma center late in the evening. I examined him, prepped him for surgery, and removed the blood clot as swiftly as I could, and the patient spent the remainder of the night in the ICU without any major issues. I updated his family on his condition and confirmed that things had gone as well as we could expect and now we just had to wait to see how he recovered. It was a routine neurosurgical case, and it was a success. I was feeling proud of myself for handling this case, for taking call while seven months pregnant. I was handling the job.

Dr. Egan wanted to make sure if this was a game, I knew I was not winning.

Everything about this Grand Rounds session started off as routine, beginning as it usually did, with a fatigued resident, black lines under his eyes, tousled hair, standing before the crowd next to a raised podium. He commenced his rehearsed presentation.

"This patient is a forty-five-year-old male with a history of headaches and gait disorder. Patient noted that he was imbalanced and began experiencing repeated falls." He paused to take a breath. I was reminded of the droning economics teacher in the film *Ferris Bueller's Day Off*. "He was fairly healthy, diagnosed with hypertension, taking a Lopressor, 25 mg daily—otherwise no surgeries, no drug allergies."

The other resident staff and attendings in the audience watched the initial CT scan as it flashed onto the projector screen. Some of the junior residents slumped in their seats, hoping to not be called upon to answer questions, not unlike that pained high school class from the film.

The radiologist attending the conference spoke next. "So, what we see here is a mass located in the posterior fossa midline, but slightly to the right. There is surrounding edema and compression of the fourth ventricle, causing hydrocephalus."

From the back of the auditorium, Dr. Egan snapped, "So, Dr. Dewan, what do you want to do next?"

I had been prepared to answer questions. This was what was expected of us neurosurgery residents: to diagnose, to plan a differential, to execute the plan.

"I would examine the patient for signs of impending neurologic decline, such as nausea or vomiting, and transfer to the ICU of present. I would place a ventriculostomy if needed and then further obtain an MRI with or without contrast-weighted dye."

Without missing a beat, he asked, "What are you forgetting?"

I ran through my algorithm of history, presentation, and plan. I visualized the diagnostic imaging. I couldn't think of what I had forgotten. "I'm not sure . . . this is what I would do initially." I trailed off.

"What about blood thinners?" he shot back. "You would place an external drain without so much as asking about blood thinners?"

"But the case history stated he was on no meds with the exception of Lopressor," I responded. Lopressor is for high blood pressure; it relaxes the blood vessels, it's not a blood thinner.

"Just . . . keep going. What would you do next?" I could hear the seething in his tone.

"I would discuss with the patient and family that this mass could represent a pilocytic astrocytoma, cerebellar metastasis, hemangioblastoma or, less likely, a glioma." I took a breath, measured my speech. "I would order a CT of the chest, abdomen, and pelvis with and without contrast to evaluate for metastasis."

He pounced like a panther. "What are you forgetting?"

I ran through my rolodex of differential diagnosis and my treatment plan. I thought back to any cases that I had with this pathology.

"Um, medications. I would start Decadron, a steroid, every six hours."

He bared his teeth. "Why would you not ask about family history of von Hippel-Lindau disorder? That is linked to hemangioblastoma of the brain. To not know that or ask if this ran in the family would leave you unprepared surgically."

"Yes, of course, I would ask about family history of VHL," I responded.

"You need to read up about VHL and give us a talk about this next week. These answers should be on the tip of your tongue."

It was then I realized I couldn't win.

I could see how excited he was to be holding all the cards firmly in his hand. His voice quickened. "What's your surgical approach?"

"I would place the patient prone in pins and make a hockey stick style incision to encompass the dimensions of the tumor. I would utilize navigation for this purpose."

"That's the most ridiculous thing I have ever heard." His voice bellowed through the room. "A *hockey stick* style incision? Where did you learn that?"

We had actually used that incision shape two weeks earlier while resecting a brain tumor in this location with these characteristics.

"The only incision to make in this case is the paramedian variety. You should know this."

Now, almost ten years in practice, I use the hockey stick style incision routinely for these tumors. But in that moment, with him holding all the power, I hung my head and said nothing more. As I left the auditorium, waddling in my scrubs, I made no eye contact with the group of interview candidates I passed.

This "Socratic display" from this attending was a clear indication for the next resident, if she was a woman: don't get pregnant in residency. That doesn't belong here.

I have always had thick skin. I have always been a strong person. But as I left that Grand Rounds session, I felt my love and commitment for neurosurgery turn brittle and crack. All because of the ugliness of some person who should otherwise have had no bearing on how I lived my life. On whether or not I had children.

After that, I had to work the full day. I hurt both bodily and to the depths of my psyche. The five minutes it took to get home felt like an hour. Alex had put Amara to sleep an hour earlier, after having kept her up past her bedtime to wait for me. I pulled myself up the stairs, my swollen feet aching, and entered her room. It was dark and smelled sweet and pure. I waddled to her crib to listen to her soft sighs and moans. To watch her chest rising and falling. She was absolutely precious, this amazing being Alex and I had brought to life, who I was responsible for loving and keeping safe and cared for. I didn't bend over to kiss her. I wanted to make sure she slept deeply.

I came downstairs and Alex had a reheated dinner plate waiting for me. I tried to hold back the welling in my eyes, but Alex saw. He always saw.

"What happened." He said it more as a statement than a question. He knew the drama that had been accumulating. He knew that my colleagues were not like his colleagues. None of mine would ever throw me a baby shower. His were once again showering us, and me directly, with advice emails, boxes of hand-me-down clothing, mildly used car seats.

I told him how the day started, the night call, and then the Grand Rounds conference. "It didn't matter what I said, Dr. Egan was determined to shame me in front of the candidates." I started to shake as I told him of my disillusionment. "How can people who save lives be so hateful toward another person giving life?" I thought back to the tone of Dr. Egan's voice, the spark of malice in his eyes. Sure, it's hyperbole, but he showed the gleam of someone who was thrilled to be humiliating a pregnant woman in front of a hundred people. Someone who dared defile his territory with her womb.

"I—I don't know, I never thought I would feel this way. I don't know if I want to go back." That was it. I said it. I said I wanted to quit the job that I had loved so deeply. I felt shattered. Is this what does it, is this what happens to women? Is this why there are so few women who are neurosurgeons? How many get mobbed out of practice by bullies? I held my belly. It was the closest to despair I had ever felt. I couldn't believe I had let a person make me feel this way. All the joy that my pregnancy had brought me on a personal level was also my weak spot. My mothering hormones were leading the charge. I had been hit in the stomach, I had put my body through hell, I had taken so much call that I was in a place beyond fatigue, and that very morning, I had felt a surge of pride, riding a tremendous high because of all that I had achieved, only to be knocked down by someone determined to see me fail. I put my head in my hands, too tired to even sob. If only I could have turned into a mother tiger, protecting her cubs, being fierce and powerful and fearsome.

I felt trapped, way past the point to turn back. What would have happened if I got a do-over? How would things have been if I had taken Door Number One and had stayed in neuroscience research? The public humiliation, the forty extra pounds I was now carrying, waddling up and down the hospital, unable even to climb a flight of stairs. I couldn't find myself anymore, and the ugliness and negativity around me made it impossible to see with any objectivity or my place in the middle of all this. Maybe I wasn't good enough for this job. It was swallowing me, and I couldn't breathe. With all the naysayers around me, all the self-doubt that had been accumulating had no seawall to keep it from swelling over. I was a failure. I had failed to become a neurosurgeon and do the thing I had always wanted to do. Maybe there was a way out, a do-over, even in general surgery, where I wouldn't be ostracized, where there would at least be other women who understood what I was going through. Even Dr. Cahill in all his wisdom and generosity couldn't guide me through this aspect of my residency. Maybe, I thought to myself then, *I haven't been giving 100 percent of myself at work, let alone the necessary 110 percent.* Maybe it was my failing all along.

Alex sat back and reflected. Then he reached over, rubbed my lower back. "Sheri, your decision to become a neurosurgeon should have nothing to do with other people. It's not about them. It's not about him. It's about you. You need to love what you do."

I sat up. "I'm not sure if I love being a neurosurgeon anymore."

Alex nodded. "You need to decide that for yourself. Look, I don't love you because you are a neurosurgeon. I love you for you. You could be a janitor cleaning the hospital floors and I would love you. You could come home smelling like a waste management plant and I would love you. Your job is only a small part of who you are."

It was true, to an extent. Hadn't I also loved neuroscience research? Not as much as I loved neurosurgery, but other surgery—of course I would make a good general surgeon. But again, PhD researcher, general surgeon, though these were lofty and noble goals, they didn't feel . . . me. Was that only because I'd devoted so many years to neurosurgery that I couldn't see beyond that?

And Alex. He had committed himself to neurosurgery as well. When he'd agreed to be my spouse, he shared the same level of commitment to help see me through my training. Alex might not have understood the full extent of that commitment when we set out, but what I have always loved about Alex was his willingness to take chances. Unlike many people who look for convenience, an easy way of life, Alex would take the leaps—his dreams, my dreams. He made that leap fully with me, never once questioning it the way many other spouses do. My residency, our commitment.

I picked at my plate of reheated food, and already the big block letters of "quit" were disappearing.

Afterward, while Alex was getting ready for bed, I called my parents. I needed their brand of advice—I wasn't taking a survey, by any means—I knew they would tell it to me straight, and they didn't have to live with the consequences of the decision in the same way that Alex would.

My dad answered the phone, as my mom was in the shower. My mom had been peppering me with motivational anecdotes over the past weeks, saying things like, "Remember Dr. Martin Luther King: 'Out of the mountain of despair, a stone of hope,'" or she would talk about the tortoise and the hare, the slow and steady being the winner. It was what she did; she motivated people with her plethora of catalogued anecdotes, and I could always rely on her for a nugget of wisdom. My father was less vocal, but he had always been supportive, nonetheless.

After I explained what happened, my dad then said, calling me *Beti*, daughter, "Never let anybody make you feel small with their words."

That was so like my dad, to drop these perfect pearls right at the moment I needed one.

"Can you do the job?" he asked.

"Yes. I think so."

"You've been doing it for six years. You know better than anyone what you can handle."

A little later, my mom got on the phone. Between the two of them, I could calm down a little more. They were my seawall against the rushing tide of negativity. My mom had been my living, breathing motivation to become a neurosurgeon. What I had needed was to hear her voice in that moment to really bring me back to my sense of purpose.

After the phone call, I got on the floor, and I meditated. I pictured what the next year and a half might look like, just as I would visualize the steps of a surgery. That night I pulled from history.

I thought of all the neurosurgeons I had read about throughout my training. Harvey Cushing, one of the founding fathers of neurosurgery, who solved the problem of excessive brain bleeding by developing a silver wire clip to control hemorrhages. Wilder Penfield, Victor Horsley, William Osler, Alexa Irene Canady, and Sofia Ionescu. How these physicians had experienced hardship but continued, pressed onwards despite the odds. How they had people who didn't believe in them but still had enough conviction in themselves that they simply didn't care what others said.

Then, I pulled from my own experiences. I thought of how I felt when patients did well, when they lived, when they thrived, when they came back to the office and hugged me and told me I had touched their lives. The patients who had kissed my hands before surgery, saying, "I hope you slept well last night." The patients who blessed me with their prayers. The patients who told me they owed me their life, despite my protests that there was no debt, that they owed me nothing. They trusted me with their very survival. How amazing to be that person to them.

I remembered an anecdote that I had read about Wilder Penfield, a Canadian-American neurosurgeon who practiced in the 1970s. He used to write letters to patients' families, even after the family member had died. Essentially a condolence card. He showed love for his patients, even after they were gone.

We neurosurgeons are so tremendously meaningful to all our patients, to their lives and their stories. I reflected on my mother and her story.

Being a neurosurgeon was about helping patients, about giving back to families what disease was trying to take. This dream of mine wasn't about attendings with an ax to grind.

I wasn't ready to walk away. If I didn't get up and go back tomorrow, there would be no going back. I would be shutting that door. Alright, so could I be this person?

The next morning, my clock beeped at 5:00 a.m., jarring me awake.

I turned onto my side, heaving up my taut belly, dangling my legs from the bed. I sat there, my hands gripping the edge of the bed, my belly a bulge that kept me from leaning forward, and I thought, *This is it. I'm all in. I'm not going to back down. I'm going to dedicate myself 100 percent to what I'm doing.*

I didn't want to use my pregnancy as an excuse. I didn't want to use motherhood as an excuse. There were no excuses.

All-in. It would become one of my primary mantras. Any time I found myself adrift, I would recommit to my moonshot goal, reaffirm that I was all in, so I *could* do this life and I *would* do this life—on my own terms.

I went into work, just like any other day. *Because I am a neurosurgeon and I'm all in.*

The days were better. I had the staff to support me, and most importantly, there was the work. I loved my job. Every minute in the operating room reminded me of my purpose. And I even got a couple of miracles.

Dr. Cahill had become not just an instructor but a mentor. He'd had my back during my pregnancy, and as I moved from junior to senior resident, his support was the exact foundation at work that I needed to keep my head straight and stay focused on the job that I loved so much.

He brought me in on a special procedure. I would be assisting Dr. Cahill in implanting a deep brain stimulator on a man with severe Parkinson's disease. I had seen patients with Parkinson's before, but not with such a profound tremor; so profound, he was tremoring off the bed and had to be restrained. Performing brain surgery on a patient with violent shaking has its own set of complications. We used the soft wrist restraints tied to the bed, then wrapped a white sheet around the patient, forming something like a papoose. Dr. Cahill was the lead, although I performed the craniotomy, then stepped back to watch Dr. Cahill expose the brain and implant the stimulator.

"Okay," Dr. Cahill said, several hours into the surgery, the magnet in place. "Let's see if this takes." He turned on the magnet, and I watched, mouth agape, as the patient's tremors eased and then were gone, as if they were evaporating into the air of the OR. I had never seen anything like it. "I'd call that a success, wouldn't you, Dr. Dewan?"

It was remarkable. The device wouldn't be a cure for the Parkinson's, but it would certainly help this patient live a better, fuller life.

"Alright, Sheri, I'll have you stitch up that dura. Nice and tight."

As I sewed the top, tough layer of membrane over the brain, watching it pulsate, I once again marveled at what we could do in this room. I was so grateful to Dr. Cahill, to Alex, to my parents, for their support. But also, I was grateful to myself in these moments, for sticking through the bad, because there would always be this. I was where I belonged.

Sometimes you are going to run up against that one wall that feels too much, the final straw, the bridge too far. That's when you have to make the decision: are you willing to give up everything you've worked for so long, so hard, already made so many investments and sacrifices to achieve it? If the answer is to give up, then it's good to know that as well, and then you can start making your new map. But if your answer is no—out of fear or because it feels all too much—take your moment to meditate and focus (the steps are all recurring). Allow yourself to be upset, and then take whatever agency you have in order to persevere. Choosing to be all in is the point where you discover there is no going back, coming to the last off-ramp possible, and making that choice to continue ahead.

I had nothing actually preventing me from performing neurosurgery. As my dad had asked, "Could I do the job?" Yes. Yes, I could. I had been doing it for nearly six full years. I did not have an injury or a disease that suddenly rendered me unable to do the work. I didn't have to make a choice between following a dream and providing for my family. The life was hard, but I reminded myself this was what I'd signed on for. And that the worst of it was going to be temporary. I remained in full control of whether or not I achieved my dream.

If you really are in control, you can find your way to yes by staying passionate, and then you get through the toughest hurdles by committing yourself to being all in. Alex would say it's similar to *The Matrix*, when Neo realizes he is The One and suddenly is capable of bending the virtual world at his will. Tell yourself this is your life. It's worth the hard parts because it's your dream. No one said it would be easy—embrace that. Let yourself grow into it. But also take time to meditate, care for yourself, and acknowledge when it does get hard so that you don't let yourself get burned out.

9

Check In and Recenter

Being all in is an important step, but you also have to remember that you aren't all in at the cost of your health or well-being. You have to take a look at where you are on your path from time to time, to make sure that not only are you on track and your strategies are still aligning with your goals, but also that you are processing what needs processing and making sure you have even a modicum of time for your needs.

When we recenter the brain, we set goals, intentions, and search for new patterns and habits. This can calm our anxieties and fears by cooling down the amygdala, the fear center of our brain. Over time, this makes us believe that we have more control over our surroundings and are the primary driver in our own fate.

Committing to my all-in plan didn't automatically make every part of my life easier. Part of being all in, even to this day, involves reminding myself that I have to stick to that commitment. I would be a neurosurgeon and a mom. I was nailing the neurosurgeon part. But there were times I felt like I was floundering as a mom.

———◇———

It was toward the end of my pregnancy with Mia when I had to plan Amara's first birthday party. In Indian culture, the first birthday is almost as big as a wedding. The first birthday represents strength in survival after the early months where infant mortality can (traditionally) be high. It marks the official entry into the family, and it represents the promise for the future.

I was not going to be giving Amara her first birthday Indian-wedding style because that would be impossible. We were going to have it at our house, with a few friends and our family, nothing extravagant. My mom had been the queen of birthday parties. When Jiji and I had our birthday parties, our mom would go all out, but not with catering or staff; she did it all herself. She made party favors by stitching little pouches out of pink and blue material and filling those with corn kernels. She made cupcakes from scratch, chocolate cake from scratch. The decorations were also perfect. I felt intense pressure to meet that expectation, those standards that I had grown up with. My mom certainly wasn't pressuring me to be an Instagram influencer with this party (though this was years before Instagram was a thing). But there was the seed of expectation planted—it is an Indian-mother thing. Indian mothers are kind and supportive but also firm in that there are expectations that need to be met. They push us to excel.

So, despite my work schedule, I mapped out time the day before Amara's party to get the cups and plates and napkins and decorations, then do some of the prep work a day ahead. I was all set to leave work when the chief resident popped into my office and said, "Cover me?" This meant he wanted me to cover his call for the night: until 7:00 a.m. the next morning, where I would need to sleep at the hospital. I looked at him and said, "Really?" I didn't divulge that I had Amara's birthday, that I wanted to prep, but it would be a sign of weakness to say I had something personal. "Look," he said, "I really need you to help me out." He wasn't trying to be a jerk about it, but there was a hierarchy. Also, he had helped me out in the past. And, as he knew, as I knew, as everyone knew, I wouldn't be taking any call when I was on my maternity leave coming up. I couldn't say no.

There was no place online where you could order and have overnight delivery. Alex couldn't do it because he was working and taking care of Amara, who was colicky at the time. The life of a neurosurgeon is one that is meticulously planned out, and then that plan gets blown up because our lives are filled with chaos and trauma, and our daily lives are filled with last-minute curveballs. I got off call at 7:00 a.m. and went home, showered, and did what I could to get ready for Amara's small party.

I felt horrible that I didn't have all the supplies the way a "good mom" should. I was trying to do it all and wasn't succeeding; I couldn't be this mom, this neurosurgeon, be pregnant, work overnight, come home, and have a perfect first birthday party. A female tiger is often the sole provider of food for her cubs, considered a super mom of the animal kingdom. I felt very far away from being a tiger in that moment.

As I was setting out regular plates, my mom, who was already offering a world of help to me, commented, "Oh, you don't have party plates?" When I said no, I hadn't been able to get away from work to get them, she said, "Well, you'll be better prepared next year." For whatever reason, that comment, though not intended to be mean-spirited, really hurt me. The queen of the birthday party had deemed that this didn't quite measure up. It was like being fileted at Grand Rounds. What had I done that was wrong? What decision did I make in one of the steps that set everything in motion for me to not get it all done and have a negative party outcome? I was trying to juggle it all, keep a clean house, and even having a nanny wasn't enough to get everything done. Despite being busy with work, my mom had always gotten everything done, and I couldn't even manage the stupid plates. It was a total Mom Fail.

Of course, my pregnancy hormones and fatigue made everything seem worse, and my mom would have been devastated if she saw that one of her offhanded comments had stung me. But this all begged the larger question: was not having cute paper plates at a first birthday party really a fail?

Societally, women put intense pressure on themselves to be perfect, and perfect in every way, whether it's how clean you keep your house, how much you're excelling at your work, how smart your children are, how well dressed the kids are, how well dressed you are, how bang-up the party is for your one-year-old while barely juggling your job, being pregnant, and having wholly unsupportive colleagues at work. This Mom Guilt that we carry seems to be different from Dad Guilt. Dad Guilt would say, "Yeah, sorry, I couldn't get there, it just didn't happen, and I'm sorry." But with Mom Guilt, you keep it in your head and don't let it go, you remember all of the times you failed your kids somehow.

It would be some time after Mia's birth that I would be able to brush off these so-called Mom Fails as not actual fails, reminding myself that I could let it go, that more often than not, I was doing something for work, I'd be operating, I'd be saving a life. I was dealing with people who arrived at the ER dead because of a massive stroke or paralyzed and unable to speak. When compared with that kind of tragedy, the minutiae really don't matter. I'd like to think I gained that healthy dose of perspective fairly quickly, but no, I didn't have that perspective the day of Amara's party.

This was all pre-Instagram, and social media competition and pressures were not pervasive in the way we see them influencing the culture today. Now, there are these beautiful pictures of celebrities and "influencers" that breed comparison. In the months leading up to Mia's birth and afterward, I wanted desperately to be a normal mom. I held out hope that after I finished training, life could be normal. I wanted to be the mom who brought her kids to school and picked them up at the end of the day, who planned birthday parties and playdates and handmade cupcakes and vegan foods. What I realized was that person was never going to be me. I could live vicariously through the stay-at-home moms I knew. It turned out, I would rely on those stay-at-home moms for advice, such as what camps were the best, or where I should take my kids for fun or for extracurricular activities. I never had the time to do that kind of research, and they did.

I wish I could go back to that frustrated, frazzled, and very pregnant Sheri feeling like she failed Amara on her first birthday and tell her that our kids don't care about super-fancy first birthday parties. All they care about is that you're there and that you're involved with their lives, in whatever way that is. I would tell her, "Your kids want you to be engaged, they want you to put away the cell phone, they want you to delegate that call to somebody else that night and just be there 100 percent for them." I think if a parent can do that, in whatever way they can, maybe that means it's not the *quantity* of time but the *quality* of time that matters.

So that was what I actively started doing and continue to do to this day. I come home, put the phone away, turn it on silent if I'm not on-call, and then be 100 percent engaged with my kids so that they know I'm there for them. When I walk through my front door, I take off that neurosurgeon hat and put on the mom hat and wife hat. When I got back to the hospital, or at least once Alex takes the kids to school, I'm a neurosurgeon again. That was the shift in thought that I needed: I couldn't be all things all at the same time. But I could be the best of all in their assigned spaces.

Even that wasn't the waved magic wand that made everything so much easier. I was in for a whole new type of culture shock of being a working mom of two kids.

There were people who said, "Oh Sheri, your second time having a baby won't be as bad. Now your body knows what to do, so birth will probably be much easier." What my body knew was that my water breaking signaled thirty hours of labor. So, when it was time and Mia's water broke, I still had another thirty hours of slow dilation and pushing and labor cramps. But then she came and was healthy and beautiful and I fell madly in love all over again.

This time around, I didn't have to learn how to do everything. I knew to check the bath temperature. I knew how to hold the baby and all the day-to-day stuff. With our nanny helping, cooking meals, taking feeding shifts so I could get some rest, things felt more in control . . . to an extent. As much as I knew what Amara needed and wanted, Mia was an entirely different being.

Amara had colic, but poor Mia had GERD—Gastro-Esophageal Reflux Disease. Every time Mia ate, she would upchuck. We'd give her milk, she'd drink about an ounce, and then she would start making this sound like Linda Blair's Regan in *The Exorcist*, and that was the sign that the vomit was going projectile. It wasn't unlike a cat hurling up a furball; we'd hear that characteristic noise and then run her to the garbage can or sink to try to aim it to a safe place. Finally, her pediatrician told us to give her Zyrtec. I put it in Mia's milk bottle that night as I fed her in bed. She took one suck of it and, like Regan, she projectile vomited all over the back of our bed. The poor thing vomited so many times a day that we took to laying blankets on the floor and over furniture like sheets because the spit up was everywhere. And our sainted nanny washed the sheets every single day. That was how we lived every day for a year.

Because of her GI upset, Mia also screamed all the time. All. The. Time. For her entire first year, until her GI system became mature enough to handle food. The pediatrician said Mia might just be one of those kids who, as she gets older, will run around and puke. (Fortunately, that didn't turn out to be the case, and as she got older, she could eat anything and had the metabolism of a racehorse.)

So, I had all the boxes checked: two healthy girls, great husband, incredible nanny, and was in the final year of neurosurgical residency. I'd made it, right? Wasn't I supposed to feel nothing but gratitude for this nearly perfect life, having achieved my goals and shown everyone that I, that any woman, could be a neurosurgeon and a mom?

Though I loved my girls and Alex and work, I was now hanging on by a thread. On the outside, all everyone saw was a calm and collected mom of two who was also a neurosurgeon at the end of her training. When I'd take the girls to the pediatrician, he would say, "God, you're such a strong, confident mother." But I had a picky eater and an eater who threw up everything she ate. I was barely getting any sleep, and that lack, which I thought I'd mastered, was a whole different beast after having two kids. I'd survived the public shaming when I was pregnant and said I was all in. I meant it. But it was really hard to live it. I knew there was a light at the end of the tunnel, but that light currently seemed unreachable.

My colleagues were still a mixed bag. Though they didn't have to look at my round belly anymore, the sheer fact of my motherhood set off an impulse of passive aggression in a few of them. Also, there were the natural ups and downs of a really intense job that was literally life and death every day. We were all prone to being uptight. Instead of lashing out at anyone, though, I kept it all in, ever the team player. I couldn't let anyone see me frustrated—again, no signs of weakness. However, that sometimes meant I'd vent my frustrations to Alex, sometimes even at Alex. I wasn't actually circling back to take out the pin and process all the difficulties. As much as I kept my emotions under wraps at work, they were far more likely to burst out if Alex and I had disagreements.

Because for the first time in our relationship, we were having disagreements.

For the first time in our relationship, we discovered we disagreed on certain crucial points, those crucial points being our kids. More specifically, we had very different styles when it came to our kids' eating habits.

Mia was still only barfing up milk, not yet to solids, but Amara, barely even a toddler, was already experiencing the brunt of Alex's family belief that you have to clean your plate at every meal. Alex was always a huge stickler about eating, about not wasting food, which stemmed back from his mother. My mom had been much softer on this topic, saying, "If you're not hungry, that's okay," and then we'd eat when we had an appetite (this didn't mean we snacked on junk in lieu of eating real meals, however). For Alex, mealtime was mealtime.

Alex had taken to glaring at Amara to make sure she finished all her food, but Amara would hold firm.

"Amara, you haven't eaten your carrots," Alex said.

Amara pursed her lips tight. She glared back. If there was a tumbleweed in the house, it would have rolled across the room at that point. Alex furrowed his brow. Amara squinted back, just as determined. I could almost hear Ennio Morricone's score hanging in the air, the high flute representing Clint Eastwood's Man with No Name.

Alex picked up a slice of carrot. "Amara, I mean it. You need to finish your meal." He pushed the carrot at her mouth. She shook her head and craned back in her seat. I wondered if I would get a page from the hospital any time soon. Maybe they would need me for something. I wanted to let Alex handle his battles, and this was one battle I couldn't get behind. It was a spaghetti western without the spaghetti, and if we were playing out our roles, I was the *Good*, and I'd let Alex and Amara duel it out for *Bad* and *Ugly*.

Then the carrot was there again at Amara's mouth. "Amara, this isn't a game. You have to eat this!"

Suddenly, Amara was screaming. There's always the moment in the old westerns when the side players have to decide if they're going to get involved, choose a side, stick out their necks and risk taking the blast. Amara's scream was that moment for me.

"That's it! Stop force-feeding her!"

"But she needs to learn to eat everything on the plate!"

"She doesn't want it! She isn't hungry! Do you think it's going to make it better if eating becomes a trauma?"

"If she learns it now, then it will become routine. It would help if you would help me enforce this."

"I can't because I don't agree with it. Why should I have to enforce your rules of authoritarian eating?"

So began the battle without end. It was the only real fight Alex and I ever had, and it would play out at regular intervals, whenever we were all at the table together. He would get upset at me for not helping him enforce the rules, and I would affirm that they were not my rules. He was absolutely dogmatic about it. My whole thought was that Amara wasn't actually a picky eater; she was quite a healthy eater and rarely had sweets. She liked the food, but when she was finished, she was finished. Her inclinations were to graze. She'd play a little bit, then eat a little bit, then come back and play. She was never going to be one of those kids who would sit down and devour an entire meal. Try as he might to reshape that habit, Alex would not succeed. Amara reminded me so much of my sister in that way: she knew what was best for her, and she was going to stick to her principles (or a two-year-old's instincts).

Maybe she, too, had a little stripe of tiger in her.

The meal would end, and the fight between Alex and I would resolve itself. We were good about not carrying our disagreements for very long. We had so many other things going on in our lives that any squabbles or grudge-carrying seemed petty. We said what we had to say, then we moved on.

The next battle: my body did not feel like my own. I'd been lucky to recover relatively well after Amara's birth. I'd worked so much as soon as I got back from my first maternity leave that all the baby weight melted off and I didn't have to think about the lethargy or the strain of the clothes that didn't fit right or the additional pain of staying on my feet for marathon hours with extra weight any longer. However, now, after the rapid fire of my daughters' births, my body didn't fully recover and now was protesting.

Shortly after Mia's birth, I became chief resident, which meant I was working as much as I ever had, and I was on-call every day—essentially, twenty-four-seven. I was missing meals while in surgery but otherwise stuck to my dietary routine; however, that wasn't cutting it. Despite my love for fitness, running, and yoga, I didn't have time to fit that into my day, nor did I even have the energy to think about working out after my shifts and calls. I was depleted. What I did have were two blessed weekends a month in which the senior resident would take over for me. Finally, several weeks after going back to work, I'd had it. I was determined to get the pregnancy weight off me and get more energy back. I needed the endorphins. I pulled out the two-seater baby jogger and put Amara in one side and sleeping Mia in the other. It was spring and warm enough to take Mia out as long as she was wrapped in a blanket and wore a hat. As I put on my running shoes and headed for the door, our sweet Australian cattle dog, Blue, looked at me with the most forlorn eyes. Blue had not been getting out much either. "Okay, fine," I said, grabbing Blue's leash. The four of us headed out.

Here I was, the lover of running, not having worked out in months, trying to run uphill while pushing two babies in a jogger, pulling on a dog who wanted to stop every few feet to smell every single one of those roses, and I was huffing and puffing. This was not the way I had envisioned this morning.

As I rounded the corner, I came upon an older woman power walking in the opposite direction. She was decked out in her Lululemon shirt and leggings, topped with the just-perfectly-matching hat, and took one look at me. "Oh, doesn't that look like fun?" I was pretty sure she was serious and not being condescending, or maybe she was trying to be sympathetic. I was sure what I was doing was not her kind of fun. I made some sort of noncommittal noise of affirmation as I huffed on, but I was annoyed. This was supposed to be my first weekend to myself, and I was trying to exercise and get off some of the pregnancy weight. I was exhausted, wrangling my dog and two babies, and I did not need her statements on my process. No, it wasn't fun. Except, when I stopped as Blue found something to urgently pee on, I couldn't help but laugh. This was funny. I'm sure I was a sight. There was hilarity in this situation of me trying to juggle all these moving parts. I reminded myself, I'm here, I'm still living and breathing with a pulse. Perspective.

I was gifted with two wonderful, healthy daughters. I was so happy to have them in this world. I thought back to the babies I had helped deliver, to knowing how babies were born all over the world, to see the disparity of life for children. There was so much Alex and I could give our children, so much we could teach them. I was fortunate to be able to juggle motherhood with my profession, with a loving and supportive husband and an amazing nanny—even though with her help, Alex and I were still overwhelmed and exhausted. I wasn't sure if I could really get back into shape. I still hesitated when I asked myself if I could really overcome all these obstacles and be a neurosurgeon and a mom.

I then had to sit myself down and remind myself that I was all in. *Okay*, I said, *I'm going to be the best wife, the best mother, and the best neurosurgeon that I can be.* It was a statement that I had to make; it was a concrete goal. Part of my personality was having that drive and motivation to set goals, to believe in myself, and then to get it done. Okay, then. Mom hat. Wife hat. Neurosurgeon hat. And a Sheri hat, one that I would use to motivate myself to do the things I wanted to do, such as get outside and run. Those were my quantifiable goals.

As soon as I made that statement, the "decision" was made. I structured the last year of my residency to schedule time for all my hats. I committed to running, serious running, and finally, the weight did come off and I physically felt better in my body. My energy and endurance increased. I committed to being a present mother and wife, and I felt more rested and relaxed at home. I committed to being the best possible neurosurgeon I could be, and I wound up pushing myself to places I didn't even think I could go. The operative skill level was on a different plane after that. Things that would have terrified me as a sixth-year resident I was now doing with ease. I surprised myself. I didn't know I had this level of ability to juggle everything within me, but I had the safety net of my training and my dedication to get it done no matter what. I could turn off the pain and fatigue because I was unequivocal on reaching and maintaining all my goals.

Part of my recentering process was deciding on my percentages. I wasn't ever going to be able to leave work completely at work, not when I had to receive phone calls with patient updates, but when I was with my kids, I could be 100 percent their mom. I just wasn't going to be the mom who did the fancy birthday parties and the extras that other moms could do. Alex and I would have our time as a couple, and I would be 100 percent his wife in those times, but we also shared our lives with our work and still listened to each other's work stories because that was important to our lives. I loved hearing Alex's stories of working with his students and the impact he was making on those young lives. We got away on occasional weekends once or twice, and we cherished that. And when I was at work, that was it—I was a neurosurgeon, who yes, perhaps saw life and my patients a little differently after becoming a mom.

———————◇———————

Work life and home life can't be completely compartmentalized, but you can commit to the role when you're present in that role, whether it's the mom or dad role, the professional role, the caretaker role, or the friend role. Being a mom did make me better at my job, but I also would never think about party plates while I was working. In fact, plates weren't going to make the cut when deciding any of my percentages. That was the balance I struck.

When you're starting out or in the early planning stages, you don't yet know how things will go, so sometimes you'll have to return to your map and make those route recalibrations. Adjust to new circumstances, get in touch with your wants, and make sure you're where you do actually want to be. When you have too many things on your plate and feel overwhelmed? Recenter, take a breath, consider each item on your plate, and decide the priorities and how much of yourself to devote to it. And then remember it doesn't matter what plates you have underneath all of that.

10

Be Prepared for Transformation

Sometimes, like a chrysalis, you will be broken down before you are reformed. No, this doesn't mean that everyone needs to go through trauma to achieve success or experience growth. If you do experience trauma, you will have to work hard to find your way of transferring its power over you to something that gives you power. Otherwise, you will be swallowed up by this trauma indefinitely.

On the upside, you will learn things about yourself you never knew would be possible. You will be better for going after your dream with a clear sense of purpose and passion, and once you reach the moon, that feeling of your feet landing on soft alien moondust, well, there's nothing else like it. You are a different person from that point on. The moon, your dream, is no longer theoretical or an abstract concept, and you won't be quite the same person you were after that moment of touchdown.

———◇———

I sat down in the call room for a twenty-minute meditation. Having forced the practice into habit, I found I got more out of each meditation session, including finding my center, clarity, and mental acuity. I ran the surgery through my head, step by step.

First step: Visualize the opening step—do the craniotomy. You know craniotomies. You could do those with your eyes closed, that's how much that's in your fingers.

Next step: Open the dura.

Next step: Access the aneurysm.

The surgery would be about five hours, and I would be on my own.

In half an hour, I would be performing my first aneurysm clip. The clip would be on the same artery as my mother's aneurysmal rupture. I had seen it performed a few times throughout my residency; any time the chief resident was clipping an aneurysm was a big show. The younger residents would line the back of the room to watch, which is how it was when it was my turn to clip.

As soon as the craniotomy was completed and I had exposed the dura, the spectators came into the room. My microscope was attached to the television monitor, which displayed my view to the observers. I heard the whispers behind me: "Sheri's the chief resident. She's about to clip the aneurysm." Someone was narrating my progress to the new arrivals. They were filled with nervous excitement for me, for themselves in what they were about to see.

All I had to do was focus on the steps. I had been over this so many times, walking it through in my mind, thinking about what Dr. Cahill had previously shown me, what I'd seen the other times when I was along that back wall. Many of the viewers were actually medical students doing their rotations and had never seen anything like this up close before. There were a couple of times I heard a young woman's voice say, "No, I'm okay, it's alright," and some muffled sounds of concern.

I tuned out their voices. I was working my metal clip toward the aneurysm. Clip it off, stop the blood flow.

Then, something hit the floor. Several shrieks and commotion. The young medical student had fainted, just at the moment I was about to place the clip, and then someone said she was seizing. During my surgery, the student was having a full-blown seizure. Someone called a code blue, and everyone around me rushed to help her. Meanwhile, I stood over this patient's open head, holding my clip. Half the room went with the young med student as she was taken out of the room for treatment once her seizure was over; half remained to watch.

No distractions now. I took a breath . . . visualized the step . . .

I placed the clip.

There it was. The circle had been completed. Dr. Johnson saving my mother, prompting me to save this woman, someone else's mother, with the same procedure. Then, I heard Dr. Cahill's voice, speaking to the other medical students and younger residents. "Okay, now watch Sheri, look at these ties. Just look at how tight her ties are, how good her sewing is. She really is my right hand in surgery."

I couldn't have glowed more if I was a piece of uranium. Dr. Cahill told these future doctors that I was his right hand. The doctor who had mentored me and supported me and defended me, now using me as an example of what to do. His right hand. I closed the wound up as perfectly that day as anyone had ever closed a craniotomy.

Step-by-step, the surgery was completed. In that moment, it didn't matter what had happened in the past, with my public shaming, with the years of anxiety and self-doubt. This was the moment I knew; I really knew. This was who I was and who I would always be.

Later, the young medical student came up to apologize to me, but I was just glad she was okay. It became a funny story after the fact, the chaos of the operating room on what was for me the most symbolic moment of my residency. The medical student was embarrassed, but I told her it didn't matter. "There will be plenty of times you feel this way. That doesn't matter if you want this life badly enough. If your health is okay, don't let anything derail you. But take the time for self-care. Make sure you are well and strong, or everything will seem so much harder." I was on a high and wanted to pour all my lessons on getting past self-doubt into her, tell her to keep going and not to give up on her dream. Maybe it helped. Maybe at least she felt that someone understood what she was going through.

I went home ready to celebrate, but instead, life was waiting for me. The second I was in the door and scooped up Mia, she promptly vomited all over me. I guess the lesson there is that the act itself should be the celebratory reward.

We did have another young woman in the residency program. I was no longer the unicorn, and I hadn't blown it for the women following. She had seen the aneurysm clipping and said how great it was. We discussed process, and she had just as much enthusiasm as I did. I thought about this a lot later that day. We were both women and we both liked neurosurgery. We didn't mind the "weirdness" because we were there to help people.

My other epiphany was that it wasn't just neurosurgeons who had to be tough or deal with the gore—everything I experienced as a neurosurgeon, there was a nurse or team of nurses working beside me. They endured plenty of the unendurable. They were the ones who bathed the hoarding woman with maggots in her hair. They dealt with just as much blood, but they often had to deal with plenty more from patient aftercare. Many of them were women, though there were plenty of male nurses, and all of them were fighting against the stereotype of nursing as a "feminine" profession. What even made nursing inherently feminine? Certainly, any trauma or surgical nurse was right at the doctor's sides, up to their elbows in the macabre. Neurosurgery was hard in terms of content, yes, but we weren't alone in our weirdness for our high repulsion threshold. It wasn't about being macho. It was a lot less lonely once I understood that.

Okay, okay. Maybe I was a little "off" in the way that all neurosurgeons are, but maybe it was also time to rethink the social norms that gendered oddness. I was going to be the odd doctor who was into brains and blood but also makeup and jewelry and high heels (when I finally got to my clinic days). I would prove that my brand of neurosurgery was feminine. I was going to be my own brand of neurosurgeon.

And I was. My last year of residency flew by, and suddenly I graduated. The ceremony was short (I was the only graduate), and Alex and Jiji were there, Jiji reiterating how weird neurosurgeons were as people (admittedly, there were some odd conversations about brains that evening), but suddenly, I was no longer a resident. I was a fully-fledged neurosurgeon and peer. I overheard more than a few attendings say, *Wow, I can't believe . . . and with two kids.* I had proved it could be done. Dr. Egan didn't have much to say, although he did offer cursory congratulations, but really, what could he say? I hoped women would go on to prove him wrong time and again in the future.

There was so much I could do with my newfound freedom. Having the options now, I felt the pull to return home to Illinois. As my girls got older, I wanted them to be able to spend more time with my parents (who would also be able to help out a considerable amount, especially now that my father had retired). Alex and I were ready for a new start.

I received a job offer in the Chicago suburbs with a group of neurosurgeons, getting the call with the offer while I was at work. Elated, I rushed home to share the news with Alex. I practically bounded through the front door, and there he was with the girls. I said, "Guess what? I just got my first job—we're moving back to Chicago!"

Then I got a better look at the scene. Alex had Mia in the baby carrier, bouncing her to try to get her calmed down at least enough to stop crying from her GERD discomfort, and meanwhile, Amara was sitting on the floor crying amid a sea of chicken nugget carcasses across the floor.

"Great," Alex said, his voice flat. "Amara refused to eat her food and threw chicken nuggets on the floor."

And that was it, that was the reaction. Oh my god, I thought, this is life. Maybe I shouldn't have come straight home. Maybe my pager would go off and I'd have to go back to the hospital. I was ready to escape, and in the process, meet up with someone who would be excited for my news. Or maybe that was just something a neurosurgeon mom had to settle without. Eventually, though, the scene calmed down and Alex was happy for me and us all as a family. Percentages.

Alex finished his postdoctoral work at Brown and immediately found a job in Chicago, and we were truly ecstatic in our new endeavors. Yes, for the first time, I knew the supreme luxury of working hours. Scheduled surgeries, no twenty-four-hour call in-house. The views on the moon were incredible. I was in every sense of the word transformed.

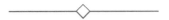

Finally achieving your dream after the long, hard grind is a truly ecstatic moment. Again, as with recentering yourself, there are no magic-wand fixes and everything in your life won't automatically be perfect. Don't put pressure on perfection, or that everyone will share in your joy in the same way; sometimes they can't, sometimes they barf, sometimes they throw chicken nuggets on the floor. However, don't let any of that stop you from marveling at the moment, at the achievement, and all that it means for you. Allow yourself the celebration, the gratitude, especially to yourself for facing all the ordeals and long hours and absolute grind. You went through all that and came out on the other end. Allow yourself the giant, bellowing-tiger roar to announce you did it.

11

———

Be Part of the Collective

Humans are not silos. What we do, what we achieve, isn't solitary. We have our most devoted lifters and supporters, our pack, the people who inspire us, the people who pick up the slack. We lean on them for help, guidance, assistance, motivation, even while we dig deep into our personal wells for strength. Tigers may be solitary creatures, but they are part of an unseen pack—the rangers and conservationists who work to protect them and their habitats. All living things are interconnected, and the world works best when everything is in harmony. Obviously, humans have the biggest impact on the environment, and there is rarely anything we achieve alone that hasn't been helped along by an entire network. Schools and teachers. Food growers. Workers at power plants keeping the lights on. This isn't meant to be a wistful, sentimental thought. I have seen the world over how much everything is interdependent: people with other people, with animals, with the land around them.

This is why it's important, when you have finally reached the point where you are able, to find a way to plug yourself back into a collective approach. What are the big and small differences you can make in the world? Can you now be, as Mr. Rogers taught us, one of the helpers? Can you share your gift and all that you've learned on your path? Can you give to others what you received along your way, or what you wished you had received?

What I bumped up against was feeling like any need for help or a break or rest was a sign of weakness. If there was one thing I would love to change about the world, it's that we don't all need to be made of Teflon, inside and out, and never have an emotional break. Yes, we need to be tough, but not 100 percent of the time (that's impossible) and so often those who act as though they are impervious end up suffering burnout, make mistakes, or end up damaging their interpersonal relationships. The inspirational memoir from neurosurgeon James Doty, entitled *Into the Magic Shop*, highlights this in a beautiful and striking way. His work was a guide to me in those years when I struggled, but what he invokes over and over is the need for acting with love and as part of a collective experience, not a self-centered one, which he learned after hard experience.

That's how I was raised. My mother's life work was about taking a look at the collective and reaching out to have not only an understanding of the economic disparities that face people around the world, but also how to do something about it. It's not about "everyone for themselves"; the world never really has been structured that way. Yet, the world is not a place of equity and justice, as it should be.

Right after my graduation from residency, Dr. Cahill brought me into his office to be awarded my graduation gift—a chair with an engraved plaque with my name and Brown University for my future office—and sat me down for a last talk. He eyed me for a moment. "This is a little something, from me." He handed me a box, and I was surprised by its weight. I unwrapped an antique stethoscope engraved with my name. It was beautiful.

"So, you are done." He cleared his throat. "I want to tell you some things about our profession that you must hear and that you must know." He leaned in, and I matched him. He had been fatherly and had given me so much advice, but we'd never had what you'd call a heart-to-heart. "We are flawed creatures, we make mistakes, we are human." He paused. Then he said, "We are also vehicles of God on Earth that have been given a very special and unique gift."

I had never known Dr. Cahill to be an overtly religious man. We affected patients' lives, but we never invoked religion; if we did, we did so sparingly. There were always patients who invoked religion, had their priests or pastors come for last rites or blessings in the ICU, but we as residents, as attendings, as surgeons, never spoke about an ethereal being that may be omnipotent and omnipresent. We never talked about *God*. Was it because it allowed for the perception of weakness? For surgeons who handled the very tissue that encompassed the sanctity of mind and spirit, why did we speak so little about these topics?

Dr. Cahill continued, "What you do with your gift is your decision. Never think about this as a job . . . or a paycheck. It's so much more than that. What you have been trained to do is so impactful."

The subtext of this conversation was: Do Good Work.

I looked away for a minute, just to blink away the tears welling in my eyes. I thought back to the night I almost left the field I cared about so deeply because of the aggressive browbeating and condescension of another person. How could I have ever believed that our profession was not important or have let an individual or group of individuals rattle my trajectory that had been decades in the making? This was, indeed, my calling.

I was sad to leave my residency. I was sad to say goodbye to my mentors who had trained me with such patience. I was sad to leave Dr. Cahill.

Mentorship in our field has unique and poignant moments. When we enter residency, we cannot suture, cannot make an incision properly, do not know how to hold a drill. At the end, we are bonified, confident surgeons. The mentor has been there throughout the process. The guide. The nurturer. The mentor has been patient and wise. The mentor can be flawed, but even in their flaws, we learn truths. Although I had a loving father back home in Illinois, Dr. Cahill had become my neurosurgical father. I had seen more of Dr. Cahill over the last seven years than I had my own father.

"Thank you, Dr. Cahill, for everything."

"It was my pleasure, Dr. Dewan."

Once I had time and bandwidth and was, essentially, my own boss, I became a mentor to young women interested in neurosurgery and worked with different organizations to promote and help women along this journey. I wanted to extend my knowledge to anyone who wanted to be a part of this wonderful, tough, weird, beautiful profession. The majority of medical students are now women, but only 5.9 percent of practicing neurosurgeons are women, according to data from a landmark paper I'd read in the *Journal of Neurosurgery*: "The Future of Neurosurgery: A White Paper on the Recruitment and Retention of Women in Neurosurgery" by Deborah L. Benzil, M.D., et. al.[1]

One of my colleagues once said, "If you see a tall tree, check how deep the roots are." Regardless of how a person defines success, when someone is achieving their goals, there are vast numbers of people who have nurtured that person along the way. There is always a supporter, a confidant, a shoulder, and inspiration at some point. I have had mine, from Alex to my parents and Jiji, to Dr. Cahill, to so many others who left their positive imprint on me.

To this day, I rely on my own network for practical advice and support. It's critical to maintain these networks to foster both friendships and lifelines. I'm a member of the group Women in Neurosurgery—an admittedly small group—but we do have a national conference, addressing advocacy for women in our field. I have travelled to various high schools, meeting with students who are interested in becoming neurosurgeons or even surgeons. At a charity fundraiser for my high school academy, I had recently auctioned off a chance for a high school student to observe me in action in the operating room, to get a taste of the kind of work I do. I have given talks at my alma mater. One student said to me, "I want to do this, but I'm worried about how the landscape of medicine is changing. What advice to you have?"

Her question was thought-provoking. The current hospital system has become increasingly corporate and bureaucratic, often marginalizing the caregivers. In so many cases, the patient doesn't come first, and outside interests determine whether the patient can receive the much-needed care. I wanted to tell her that if you love what you do, it shouldn't matter, but I also realized that was a privileged point of view. Not everyone can afford the grueling years of training for a career path that may box you out at the end. Because of this, I worry that medicine may not attract the best and the brightest for the simple fact that personal costs may be too high. More than ever, then, women need to be each other's tree roots; we need to support and lift up one another to fight for every opportunity.

I had witnessed disparities firsthand while treating pediatric patients both at Brown and at Cook County Hospital. These experiences led me to work with a foundation that supports foster children who have been through the Chicago and Illinois's housing system, often with four or five or even six different foster families. Rather than age out of the system and disappear, they can live in a freestanding facility the foundation runs, in which they staff their own teachers and school. These foster kids, who have been bounced around so much, often have behavioral problems. A therapist is on staff to help them modify behaviors, to help them cope with what they've been dealt, and to give them skills to navigate the rest of their life from that point on. There was an opportunity for me to serve on the board, and I jumped at the chance. I helped raise money and awareness. Of course, the problem is bigger than any one foundation can solve, but it is my mission to keep fighting to give as many people as possible a chance at a thriving life. I'm still fighting for those small miracles.

To fully achieve all of my goals, I found my way to doing charitable surgeries in India (despite the PhD neuroscience researcher I worked for all those years ago who didn't believe I ever would). Life had become life—it was manageable, and I felt the call to help, to do something in the world, as my parents taught me, to do good, as Dr. Cahill said I needed to do with my gift.

There are only 3,500 neurosurgeons in India, a country of 1.5 billion people. The ratio of doctors is less than one for every one thousand people—and that's doctor, not surgeon.

I was contacted by a charity private hospital in Kochi, Kerala, that was reaching out to surgeons of Indian descent to come perform as many surgeries as possible during a two-week period. I responded to the email, and they arranged for us to meet for dinner in downtown Chicago. Over the course of the next nine months, I was in touch with their department to figure out an ideal time and then arrange for all the paperwork I would need to perform charity surgeries in a foreign country.

I looked out the airplane window as we descended into Cochin, and for a moment, I was breathless. Southern India seemed awash with lush trees bejeweled with yellow laburnum flowers. The vibrant colors ran riot, and as I disembarked, the smells perfumed the air around me, so dense I could swim in it.

I only had a day to settle in before I was brought to the hospital. The intensity was, I won't say overwhelming, but I found myself pushed to the very limits of what I could do, mentally and physically. The day I arrived, there were 170 patients stuffed into the waiting room, patients of all shapes and sizes, with families and young children, dressed in traditional sarongs. Many men bore cranial injuries that were noted, skulls that had been caved in. One wife carried around her husband's fully catheted urine bag as he walked. Some, I learned, had traveled eight-to-ten hours by bus and train to be seen by a surgeon that day. Most of them spoke Malayalam, a South Indian dialect that is separate from Hindi. There are commonalities, but I struggled to understand them and was really only able to communicate with the help of one of the nurses or assistants.

I was no stranger to the struggles of access, of poverty and economics; my mother had seen to it that I had a keen knowledge of the class disparity throughout India, especially compared with places such as the United States. Seeing it, working within that system, that was the shock. The first operation I performed for was to remove a large brain tumor from a woman. The operating room was hot—there was no air conditioning in the building at all. Already I was sweating. This was how these surgeons operated on a daily basis, in the sticky heat. Who knew how sterile the room was, although everything looked clean. But there were plenty of ways incidental bacteria could have been introduced to the environment and then proliferated.

I scrubbed in, gowned, and gloved. I moved to take out the second pair of gloves—in the US, surgeons double-glove for any surgery in order to prevent any injury related tears in the latex material. If for some reason a drill or a scalpel were to penetrate the first set of gloves, the surgeons are protected by the second set.

The tech looked at me, almost breaking scrub to stop me with her hand. "You want a second set of gloves?"

"Well, that is what we normally do . . . ?" My voice trailed up into a question, slowly realizing that I was in a completely new world of performing surgery.

"One pair of gloves," she said. They didn't want to waste the limited resources they had on doubling up. Okay, I would be very, very careful around all sharp objects here.

After removal of the tumor, as I was closing her scalp, I threw the first of the pop-off sutures. Typically, in the US, we use these pop-off sutures, in which we throw the first stitch and then pop off the needle and tie. Closing a scalp flap to the degree I had done for this woman's brain tumor removal, I would probably use between twenty or thirty of these sutures.

After I popped off that first stitch to tie down the first suture, I put out my right hand for the scrub tech to hand me the next stitch.

"No, no, no. I'm sorry," she said.

I looked at her.

"We only use one stitch. More is a waste of thread."

That was it. I had to close a craniotomy with a single stitch. For every patient.

I was seeing it with my own eyes, but I still couldn't believe it, how underserved these people were, how little resourced and funded. I couldn't fathom how successful surgeries were performed in this way. And then I realized that for these patients, what I was doing for them, the access they had during this charity, it was more than they could have imagined. It hurt my heart.

I noticed one woman who carried around her child. Every time I passed the hallway, she had her child in her arms. I spoke with her in Hindi, and her son, who was almost nine years old, had cerebral palsy he developed at his premature birth, when he suffered an anoxic brain injury. His movements were spastic. Because of lack of access and economics, he didn't have a wheelchair. She had brought him all the way from their home in Northern India to ask whether her son would ever be able to walk. In the United States, he would have had a case manager, a motorized wheelchair, and significant access through the hospital. In the United States, he could have had a medication pump implanted to control his spastic movements. This mother was willing to do whatever it took to help the son she loved. The only thing that could be offered her was a one-time decompression of his nerves, to release some of the retraction and rigidity in his arms. I would only be able to do one follow-up during my stay. It's frustrating to know how little help is available around most of the globe for people like this boy whose mother was so desperate to help him live a good life.

Something was creeping through my body, something along the lines of enlightenment. The movement, though, was more like a reaching out, truly a sense of connectiveness.

I was hot, exhausted after so many surgeries in such a short amount of time, and though I was renewed by my ability to provide a little help, I was heartsore that it was so little. India was a clear display of the ongoing global health crisis. How could we live in a world with so much disparity, even among Indians? Are we really all that different? We may have different cultures throughout the country, speak different dialects of Hindi, have a range of skin tones, but doesn't this mother love her son the same way I love my children? Isn't her concern the same human emotion across the world? I decided then to make it the ongoing work of my life—I would treat as many people as I could, serve my patients with all of my power, and try to find ways to ensure that patients across the world would have access to the best treatment the world had to offer.

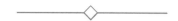

Acting communally means doing works of service and sharing what you've learned. I did this by doing both charitable surgeries and mentorships. Humans are nurtured by connectivity, by feeding the soul. We can have all the accomplishments checked off on our resumes, but the questions that follows next are: What do those accomplishments actually mean? What is the greater force or entity they're serving?

Being part of a community also means not being afraid to ask for help. In medicine, we do this all the time. We need other eyes sometimes, we need nurses and assistants, we need second opinions. Medicine by its very nature is collaborative, and it's harmful to act as if it's not. I am hard-pressed to even come up with any field of work or study that isn't in some way collaborative or communal, something that is done in complete isolation. Society functions because of all its members, and if we can help everyone to be meaningful contributors by keeping them healthy and educated and inspired, then we do nudge our world closer to something like harmony.

12

———

Sink into Success

Saying a person is "successful" is a somewhat arbitrary benchmark, as it is a highly subjective term. One person's definition of a success is a hedge fund portfolio, another's might be making it through high school or college, other people are just trying to get through the day with food on the table. What is important is that you create your own criteria for success, based on the vision you mapped out when you set out on your path. You can change your mind along the way about how far you want to go, or what you're really capable of reaching (more than you thought or sometimes less than you thought) but take your mapped path seriously throughout the process, treating it as something concrete and meaningful. Then, similar to allowing yourself to be transformed, allow yourself to feel the success of accomplishing your achievement. Continue to let the success—the whole process of getting to your success, really—be meaningful.

It's easy to get sucked into the trap of one goal never being enough and rushing after the adrenaline of chasing the next dream. If that's really where you want to be and what fulfills you, then go ahead, but again, be aware of the trap of the chase. Instead, be present for a while with your success. This is where meditation is critical. Slow the pace of life when you can (especially if you have a stressful career in which it seems impossible to slow down—trust me on this one!). Reflect, be mindful. This is where you find both your heart's desire and what matters most to you.

Look, too, for those moments when you realize you may have come full circle, armed with the knowledge of a path well cut. Allow again for the ups and downs of life, as success isn't a cure-all for all your problems or a shield from hardship. Finding the touchstone moments can help you appreciate the hard work you've done, and help you put your work into a greater context.

———————◇———————

I had been back in Chicago for two years, working at the private practice in the Chicago suburbs. We had been busy, covering several hospitals throughout Illinois and Wisconsin. Now, I was about to take a new position, moving to employment within a new hospital system.

I was on my Bluetooth with a senior colleague from the hospital as I drove from our private practice office to another hospital for a surgical consult. We were discussing hospital contract negotiations.

"It's a great hospital, the people are wonderful. You are really going to like it," he continued. I had known the hospital well, though it had been years since I was intimately familiar with it. "Oh, I almost forgot to mention," my colleague said. "I heard that one of their neurosurgeons just died, I wonder if you knew him."

"Which one?" In our field, the numbers were small; we all knew of one another in some way, either by reputation or from a conference, or had known someone who had trained with them or had been mentored by them.

"It was Dr. Johnson. Doug Johnson."

I gasped. I moved into the extreme right lane on the highway and attempted to compose myself. "When? How?"

"He just died not that long ago. It was gastric cancer, they say he went quickly."

I hung up with my colleague and eased the car off the highway, turning onto a side road to make a complete stop. I turned off the ignition. How could this be?

I had seen Dr. Johnson only one time after my mom's aneurysm follow-up appointment, when I briefly bumped into him at a surgery conference twelve years later. At the time, I was struck at how unchanged he seemed over those twelve years—he was energetic, vibrant, alive, and glowing. We were in a lecture, and as I looked around the room, I suddenly recognized the bald head and the bowtie. My heart raced at seeing him. There I was, almost a full-fledged neurosurgeon, a chief resident, in that very room in large part because of him. The previous time I saw him, I was a tentative and worried young adult. He was a few rows away from me, so as soon as the talk completed, I elbowed my way through the crowd of black and navy suits and Italian leather shoes in order to reach him.

Dr. Johnson turned and was walking toward me. He exuded excellence, strength, and power.

I shook his hand as I had that night after my mother's craniotomy. "Dr. Johnson, we have met before. You operated on my mother several years ago."

His eyes sparkled. I was unsure if he remembered her, but then he said, "Of course, I remember your mother. How is she?"

"Well actually, she retired after the aneurysm rupture. But she's well and has two grandkids that keep her busy."

"Well, congratulations to you . . . and her." He smiled. "Where are you now?"

"I'm finishing up residency at Brown, and then heading back to the Windy City come the summer."

"That's great news, there are good people in Chicago. Look me up when you get back."

"I will. I definitely will." I smiled, knowing there wasn't much more I could say at the moment. My head buzzed. "It was great to see you again."

"Likewise, take care." We shook hands one last time.

That was only a few years ago.

I had never reached out to him upon returning to Chicago, even though I had told him I would. It had often been on my mind, but life had become infinitely busy, especially after the birth of my son—a surprise third pregnancy. Now, I was signing on to work at the very hospital where he had worked, where my mother had her surgery, the place where I was inspired to become a neurosurgeon. I had hoped to see him as a colleague, had planned to work alongside him in a matter of months.

That night I called my parents.

"Bless his heart, that poor man," my mother said. "God gave him a gift. He did God's work."

My father was equally affected, though as was his custom, he contained his emotions, listening silently to my mother and me. But I knew him well enough. The news brought back so many memories of a time twenty years past, the very worst time of our lives.

I hung up the phone, my heart heavy with regret. Regret that I had never said the words to Dr. Johnson that I should have, that I couldn't say to him at my mother's last appointment, that I couldn't say at the conference, and that I hadn't said over the last few years, every one of the times I could have called but didn't because it slipped my mind or wasn't the "right" time. What I should have said was, "Thank you for your dedication. Thank you for your commitment. Thank you for all the sacrifices you made in your own life to get to the level you are now. All the sacrifices you made in your own life to serve the lives of others. Thank you for taking care of my mother. From the bottom of my heart, Dr. Johnson, you touched my life. I am forever grateful."

I thought of him as I went to bed that night, and again the next morning. I thought of him as I signed my contract, as I prepared to start my new job at the hospital, as I drove in for my first day.

I had not set foot at that hospital since I was twenty-three. Now, I was thirty-seven and a full-fledged neurosurgeon, three kids in tow. Alex and I went in a day early so I could set up my new office—I needed help bringing in my Brown graduation chair, after all.

I unloaded a box of mementos and pictures, including the picture I took of Mount Everest when my mother and I flew past it on our trip in 1999—a mountain I knew I would never be able to climb physically, though I'd summited my own Everest. A small statue of Ganesha, the Hindu god in the form of an elephant, the remover of obstacles, and typically the god Hindus pray to before examinations or major tests. To achieve the highest level of effectiveness, symbolically, I placed him on a shelf facing east. On my bookshelf, I set Dr. Cahill's antique stethoscope. Alex handed me a large gift bag. "This is very special. I found it at a local art fair, and I knew you would need it for your new office." It was a painting on a twenty-four-inch-wide canvas of a brain.

"You got me brain art?" I laughed, hard, and even harder when he pulled out the picture hooks and the hammer to hang it up.

That night, my parents came over for dinner with us, the girls, and now our surprise son, Jai, who was almost a year old. We had been happy with our two girls, and we were even somewhat overwhelmed trying to manage taking care of them with our careers. At the private practice where I had been working for a year, I was nervous when telling them that I would be taking maternity leave. I was no longer a resident at the mercy of the attendings, and I didn't have a chairman to answer to, but still. I didn't know what their reactions would be. I reminded myself that this time I was holding the cards, and I already had great autonomy. What I got was no reaction. It was as if I mentioned we got another dog. My senior partner said, "Okay," when I told him I was pregnant and would be taking off four weeks after the birth. That was pretty much it. The office staff weren't overtly congratulatory in the way of my Portuguese staff back in Providence, but they also weren't hostile or even annoyed. My pregnancy was a nonissue. It just wasn't the type of workplace to get excited about a baby and ready to throw a bunch of baby showers, but mostly because it would never occur to them to do so.

My first day, I was called down from my office to see a patient in the ICU. As I walked down the halls of the ICU, it all rushed back to me. The smells were the same. The hospital staff uses a type of wet wipe preloaded with soap to bathe patients, that scent lingered from a time long ago.

Suddenly, I was twenty-two again, smelling the wipes that the staff had used to bathe my mother. I couldn't remember her room number, but I remembered the corridor and its proximity to the family waiting room. All my memories were triggered, as was my sadness, the pit in my gut that was a visceral reaction, but I reminded myself that this was a joyful return to the hospital where I had felt so helpless. I would never be helpless and lost. Saving patients was in my hands now, in my power. I had beaten that lost feeling, just as Dr. Johnson had helped my mother beat back her neurologic disease. I was about to perform surgery in the same ORs he had.

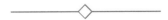

Having memories of the past and confidence for the future are all the parts of sinking into success. There is no one end goal, not with work, not with an endeavor. The work, the uphill battles, the fall downs, and the climbs back up, those are ongoing parts of existing on earth. You allow all of that to happen, to be a part of your life, your success. Success doesn't mean always fixing everything; it means learning and doing better and incorporating that at each and every turn.

Being part of the collective means true success comes when we serve as a beacon for others to achieve their goals and dreams.

Epilogue

Preparing for my present surgical case, I reviewed my patient's chart and looked over the MRI scans on my computer. I went over my surgical plan, and I drank my small bottle of cranberry juice. I stretched out my legs and began my presurgical meditation, wherein I envisioned each step of the surgery. Eight hours, but each step is a bite, and all I have to do is follow the process I know. I channel the tigress, who reacts by instinct. I've willed instinct into my hands and fingers. Even tigers, when they're cubs, are taught to hunt. We all have to learn our own way.

I cannot save every life. What I can do is offer hope and dignity. When I can save someone, pull someone out of the grip of death, that is miraculous, it is a superpower. Even if every patient were to forget me, it wouldn't matter as long as I had given them back to their families, let them lead the lives they were destined to lead.

For the ones I can't save, I can give them a moment of grace and ease their pain, let them live out their last precious time with the dignity that all human beings deserve. Though I can't help every person who needs help, I have to focus on the individual saves. Each person is important to somebody. Each person is worth saving; I just take the saves one at a time. Then I can help the next one. Then the next.

This power is a special gift I have been given, and my destiny is to share that with as many people as I can reach.

When it was time, I walked down to the operating room, *my* territory, smelling the bleached halls as I moved through the flickering fluorescent light. I was calm, though I had the electric charge I get every time I head into surgery. I scrubbed my hands with the strong antibacterial soap, in between my fingers and up to my arms. The nurse draped and gloved me, then tied the mask around my face. We pushed through the swinging doors, and there was my patient, draped and ready for my work.

All the smells were familiar, comforting. The beeps of the machines. The chill of the climate control. The tools laid out on the tables, as they should be, as they always are. The surgical crew, coordinated, awaiting my cue to start. I stepped up to the table, examined the point for my first cut, and held my right hand out for the scalpel. The weight of it as the nurse placed it in my hand, the cool grip of the metal. This, the operating room, the work, the intricacies of the human brain—this all was my home.

My heart let out a roar.

I was all in.

End.

Notes

Chapter 1

1. John F. Kennedy, "Address at Rice University on the Nation's Space Effort," John F. Kennedy Presidential Library and Museum (12 September 2019). https://www.jfklibrary.org/learn/about-jfk/historic-speeches/address-at-rice-university-on-the-nations-space-effort

Chapter 2

1. Kennedy, "Address at Rice University."

Chapter 6

1. "Tiger Fact Sheet," PBS, Public Broadcasting Service, (4 June 2020). https://www.pbs.org/wnet/nature/blog/tiger-fact-sheet/
2. "Neuroscience in Ancient Egypt," UCL, Researchers in Museums Neuroscience in Ancient Egypt Comments, (21 February 2018). https://blogs.ucl.ac.uk/researchers-in-museums/2018/02/21/neuro-science-in-ancient-egypt/comment-page-1/

Chapter 7

1. Paulette Light, "Why 43% of Women with Children Leave Their Jobs, and How to Get Them Back," *The Atlantic*, (19 April 2013). https://www.theatlantic.com/sexes/archive/2013/04/why-43-of-women-with-children-leave-their-jobs-and-how-to-get-them-back/275134
2. Claire Miller, "The Gender Pay Gap Is Largely Because of Motherhood," *The New York Times*, (13 May 2017). https://www.nytimes.com/2017/05/13/upshot/the-gender-pay-gap-is-largely-because-of-motherhood.html

3. Nitin Agarwal, Michael D. White, Susan C. Pannullo, and Lola B. Chambless, "Analysis of National Trends in Neurosurgical Resident Attrition," *Journal of Neurosurgery*, (23 November 2018). https://the-jns.org/view/journals/j-neurosurg/131/5/article-p1668.xml

Chapter 11

1. Deborah L Benzil, Aviva Abosch, Isabelle Germano, et al., "The future of neurosurgery: a white paper on the recruitment and retention of women in neurosurgery," *National Library of Medicine*, (September 2008). doi: 10.3171/JNS/2008/109/9/0378. PMID: 18759565

Acknowledgments

Writing a novel is truly a labor of love that has taken me close to four years for completion. I would like to thank my biggest supporter, my husband Alex. Without him, this work would not be possible.

My children Amara, Mia, and Jai were a source of inspiration during the writing of this book; may they have endless opportunities to cut their own path in the world.

I thank my parents for allowing me to share their story of hope and determination, and my sister, Priya Dewan Doty, who always encouraged and supported me throughout my life.

I would also like to thank my literary agent, Coleen O'Shea, who tirelessly worked to find this manuscript a home, as well as the editors and publisher who worked to finalize the manuscript.

I thank my patients for the privilege to take part in their stories and touch their lives. As well as the mentors that trained me with dedication and patience. I hope that my story can inspire many other dreamers like myself to achieve their goals using the power of purpose, discipline, and self-determination.

About the Author

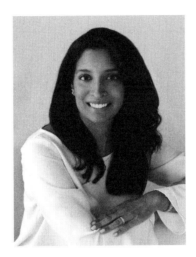

Dr. Sheri Dewan is a full-time, board-certified neurosurgeon practicing in the metro Chicago area, affiliated with Northwestern Medicine. She is one of roughly two hundred board-certified women neurosurgeons in the United States. She completed her neurosurgery residency at Brown University and graduate degree at Northwestern University. She is a proud board member of Women in Neurosurgery (WINS), Congress of Neurological Surgeons, and American Association of Neurological Surgeons. Dr. Dewan donates her time performing charity surgery in Southern India and sits on multiple charity foundation boards. She is also currently studying business and finance at the University of Oxford Executive Education program in London, England. Dr. Dewan is trilingual and has lived in five countries. In her spare time, she enjoys traveling, yoga, and spending time with her husband and three children.

Follow Dr. Dewan on Instagram @drsheridewan, or visit her website www.DrSheriDewan.com.